CENTENNIAL

WINNIPEG

JAN 13 2003

PUBLIC LIBRARY

WITHDRAWN

D1534277

CENTENNIAL

# Manmade Breast Cancers

# MAN

# CAN

# ZILLAH EISENSTEIN

# MADE
# BREAST
# CERS

CORNELL UNIVERSITY PRESS • *Ithaca and London*

*Copyright © 2001 by Cornell University*

All rights reserved. Except for brief quotations in a review, this book, or parts thereof, must not be reproduced in any form without permission in writing from the publisher. For information, address Cornell University Press, Sage House, 512 East State Street, Ithaca, New York 14850.

First published 2001 by Cornell University Press
First printing, Cornell Paperbacks, 2001

Printed in the United States of America

*Library of Congress Cataloging-in-Publication Data*

Eisenstein, Zillah R.
    Manmade breast cancers / Zillah Eisenstein.
        p. cm.
    Includes bibliographical references (p.   ) and index.
        ISBN 0-8014-3862-4 (cloth)—ISBN 0-8014-8707-2 (pbk.)
    1. Breast—Cancer—Political aspects. 2. Breast—Cancer—Social aspects. 3. Feminism. I. Title.
    RC280.B8 E375 2001
    362.1'9699449—dc21

                                                    00-011436

Cornell University Press strives to use environmentally responsible suppliers and materials to the fullest extent possible in the publishing of its books. Such materials include vegetable-based, low-VOC inks and acid-free papers that are recycled, totally chlorine-free, or partly composed of nonwood fibers. Books that bear the logo of the FSC (Forest Stewardship Council) use paper taken from forests that have been inspected and certified as meeting the highest standards for environmental and social responsibility. For further information, visit our website at www.cornellpress.cornell.edu.

Cloth printing          10 9 8 7 6 5 4 3 2 1
Paperback printing      10 9 8 7 6 5 4 3 2 1

*For Julia, and the part of her story not told here*

# CONTENTS

# PREFACE

Breast cancer is a political site from which I uncover the silences used to construct women's bodies. I share pain and suffering not simply to authenticate this way of knowing, but to push elsewhere. I do not mean to universalize from my body but rather to build a bodily history with its politics, beyond itself. I share my family story not as melodrama with victims and sadness but as a rich location for a personally passionate politics that includes the wider environments of breast tissue. I build a story that unravels and opens up with unclear markers of beginning and end.

I write in order to see what is not easy to retrieve immediately. I write of my body to discover its politics through its own specific history. I write with an urgency to turn the political agenda across the globe toward the health of the breast. I use my body's story to restart, again, the ongoing project toward antiracist feminisms that can challenge exploitation and degradation across the globe.

I want to create a more complex understanding of breast cancer. In this telling, genetics is important but not in some obvious sense. Nor is this most often the real story that needs telling. As well, the environment is important in my construction, but here too I think of environments as plural and as entering the body. We need to complicate science and its methods so we can decontaminate it.

I do not write as a scientist of the breast. I write instead as a feminist theorizing breast cancer in the hope of understanding it, and with it, our world. Theory is a way of seeing connectedness—of the breast to the rest of the body; of the body to the rest of its environments; of the historical process over time, which triggers cancer mutations, to the fluidity of borders between the breast and all else. Theory allows me to see beyond singularity and inevitability.

My kind of theory asks you to multiply your vision of things, asks you to proliferate the way you see, which multiplies the potential for think-x ing and acting. I ask you to look for what is not easily in view, which means looking for the processes of how things happen. Such theory allows a continual opening up of the realms of what is knowable and visible. In this way, the lack of total knowledge is not inhibiting but becomes part of the process of discovery and action.

As you read, use the discomfort I try to create in my language for your own discovery of what is seeable. I attempt to create openings for our viewings so that we can name the power-filled environs of a medical and pharmaceutical economy.

I want to deal more inclusively with the health of the breast and its body. Breast cancer is my crucial lens for doing this. This relationship between breast health and breast cancer is similar to the relationship between reproductive rights and abortion. Each is deeply tied to the other member of its pair, but the broader, more inclusive understanding of both breast health and reproductive rights should not be reduced to any one specificity.

I begin with the breast and end with the globe *and* I start with the globe and end with the breast. This is because the issues and the tissues of the breast are porous and seepage goes inside out and outside in. So there is no simple local or global site while each of us starts with our own body. In this instance, the globe is merely an abstraction from the body.

My travels build a theorized journey from my body to a politics of bodies for a healthful globe. The breast is never an isolated starting point because it is always already culturally and psychically filled with meanings. The detection and treatment of breast cancer are never merely scientific. Culture inflects science in treatment protocols, which change along with cultural shifts. For women who are unable to afford screening, breast cancer is as economic as it is genetic. For women of color, breast cancer is as much a part of the racism they live daily as it is a disease of women.

I am humbled by the pain and grief and terror breast disease creates. I use this pain to push beyond the dominant narratives of nonseeing and silence. Breast cancer provides both the political site and the personal lens on that site for me.

# ACKNOWLEDGMENTS

This book, more than any other I have written, was made possible by my many extraordinary friends, incredible colleagues, and disparate networks of people—some of whom I first met through this project—who shared their expertise and encouragement in wonderfully generous ways. Several of the people who assisted me in this writing have done so through each of my books, again and again.

I want to recognize the significant literatures on race and gender and feminism of the last quarter century that have been an integral part of my thought process. Much of this work provided jump-off points for this book even if it is not directly discussed as such.

In the earliest stages of this project I contacted several writers of the body for assistance in this new terrain. Louise de Salvo was of incredible help to me at this time.

As I waded into the waters of scientific inquiry and issues of public health, Nancy Krieger, of the Harvard School of Public Health, readily shared her insightful work with me. Banoo Parpia of the China Health Project at Cornell University may not truly recognize how her enthusiasm allowed me to venture forth. Her fact check helped expedite the book as a whole. Susan Snedeker and Carmi Orenstein of the Program on Breast Cancer and Environmental Risk Factors in New York State were also very helpful with my earliest queries. Cancer researcher Noa Noy of Cornell University was always ready to explain the science to me.

I wish to express my deep gratitude to Andrea Martin of the Breast Cancer Fund and Ngina Lythcott of the Mailman School of Public Health at Columbia University for speaking with me and generously sharing crucial ideas. Cindy Pearson, director of the Women's Health Network, was an extraordinary resource. Jean Hardisty of the Women's

xii  Community Cancer Project was generous with her time and assistance. Thanks also to Margaret Ratner of the Cuba Project, "Share Hope." I as well want to recognize the important local work of the Ithaca Breast Cancer Alliance.

Writings by and exchanges with Nawal El Saadawi, Chandra Mohanty, bell hooks, Meera Nanda, and Leila Ahmed helped me travel outside myself in significant ways.

Miriam Brody, Rosalind Petchesky, and Patty Zimmermann all read the earliest drafts of the book. As always, their tireless commitment to reading, and commenting, and searching with me for new ways to think and speak goes beyond the usual to the truly miraculous. Patty pushed me to be forthcoming but not melodramatic; Ros insisted on clarity and precision that I could not always deliver; Miriam read parts of the last draft with her keen and loving eye for language.

Anna Marie Smith, Mary Jacobus, Chandra Talpade Mohanty, Mary Katzenstein, bell hooks, Mary Ryan, Rebecca Riley, Ellen Wade, Carla Golden, and Susan Buck-Morss all read sections of the book and shared their thoughts with me. Their ideas and friendship are present throughout. Bell kept pushing for an inclusive title; Anna Marie for sexual openness; Chandra for a sense of creative politics.

My medical doctors have also been enormously important to this project. Katherine Husa (gynecology), Charles Garbo (oncology), and Rob MacKenzie (surgeon) have assisted both my mind and body. I want to thank especially the staff at Dr. Garbo's office for their decade-long friendship, especially Nancy Brand, Kelly Seaman, and Joan Denmark who is the only technician that has mastered my veins. Friend and nutrition specialist Victoria Wood developed the nutritional protocols I followed during chemotherapy, and continue to follow. She has also designed my daughter Sarah's nutritional program. Dr. Asa Yancey, my mother's surgeon, was kind enough to respond to each and every one of my inquiries for the book. Dr. Jill Nation, my sister Giah's oncological surgeon, became a part of our inner circle as Giah fought to live. My friend Lisa Andersen, an oncological gynecologist, assisted me through every step of Giah's protocol.

Robin Ostfeld of Blue Heron Farm provides me with the organic xiii food that my family eats, and brings me some peace of mind.

Sarah Dean assisted me with her computer knowledge, and Donna Freedline helped me through an outrageous amount of correspondence necessary to the project. Many thanks to them both.

Donald Dowsland gets special thanks for helping me find my chemo wigs and for never allowing me to stay with rigid constructs of gender for too long.

I also wish to give thanks for my incredible group of students at Ithaca College, who keep me probing and wondering about new horizons to open up and challenge. A very special thanks to Carlos Perkins, Bruce King, Rob Shainess, and Melanie Nowling. Also, special thanks to my colleagues Tom Shevory, Peyi Soyinka, Asma Barlas, Naeem Inyatalluh, and Aida Hozic in the Department of Politics, who support new trajectories of thought readily and with curiosity, and to the provost's office at Ithaca College, especially Jim Malek, who has been very generous with financial assistance for much of the work necessary to this book.

I am lucky to have met my editor at Cornell University Press, Catherine Rice, who knew exactly what this project was about before I did. Her excitement and support have been profoundly significant and have eased the entire process. Thanks to the special touch of my copyeditor, Susan Tarcov, and manuscript editor, Ange Romeo-Hall.

My community of intimate friends spread around the country and world made it possible for me to sustain much of what I write about here. They know who they are: thank you is hardly sufficient for what they allow me to continue to believe in and trust, but thank you to Ellen Wade, Miriam Brody, Chandra Talpade Mohanty, Uma Talpade Mohanty, Mary Ryan, Rebecca Riley, Zarana Papic, Patty Zimmermann, Bobbie Celeste, Randy Suzanne Ryan-Dalston, Gloria Watkins, a.k.a. bell hooks, Susan Buck-Morss, Mary Katzenstein, Sandra Greene, Carla Golden, Mary Jacobus, Anna-Marie Smith, and Rosalind Petchesky.

My daughter Sarah Eisenstein Stumbar is present throughout the manuscript, and our life together speaks for itself. I thank her for allow-

xiv ing me to share so much of her experience in such public form. My beloved partner Richard Stumbar is less present in the writing, but is my sustenance. My mother, Fannie Price Eisenstein, remains my life force. And to my sister Julia Price Eisenstein, to whom this book is dedicated, I wish life offered a second body.

This book is a testament to the way ideas are richly blended and shared, but I alone stand responsible for the way I have chosen to argue the issues of the breast.

Personalizing the Political

# Familial Breast Cancer Bodies

**B**ODIES ARE ALWAYS PERSONAL IN THAT EACH of us lives in one in a particularly individual way. They are also always political in that they have meanings that are more powerful than any one of us can determine. Femaleness, color, beauty, health are carved on us without our choice. We walk in the world trying to be seen through our own eyes while never ever fully able to do so. Breast cancer is one more challenge.

I want to go deeply into my body's story, which is entwined with my mother's and sisters' bodies. Writing my body, as feminist poet Adrienne Rich might say, allows me to think through my body to find the larger relations of power without forgetting the heartfelt intimacies. This story is not one of victimhood or melodrama. It is rather life as it is lived: the powerlessness of each of us contrasted with the enormous ability to fight back, even as we die.

2    I want to open up politics to the pain and suffering of the body and humanize the world through this journeying. So I write about breast cancer in order to demand a more just world free of the wars in iraq, kosovo, belgrade, rwanda, and pakistan and inside u.s. prisons where bodies are not taken seriously enough.[1] This is all of one piece; a politics from the breast that continues outward.

For me, my family story is not simply a personal narrative. It is not only because my family has suffered breast cancer that I have a particular critical stance toward the cancer wars and the race for the cure. It is also that I was raised, as a daughter of communist parents, with a healthy skepticism that individuals can successfully struggle alone against social problems that are rooted in consumerist profit-making institutions. I was brought up to be wary of oversimplified explanations, such as it is our genes that cause cancer, as well as skeptical of false hopes that individuals can live in isolation from their economic surroundings. So I was hesitant from the start to believe that genes, in and of themselves, can cause cancer or that one can escape the harmful societal impact of environmental contaminants that leach into our water supply and poison the food chain.

My parents nurtured us to have a strong sense of self, but I also knew that I had larger responsibilities that went beyond my own personal needs. My life was not just my own to live. I was accountable to my family and its political commitments to economic and racial justice. I was expected to be more than a selfish individual, and yet it was most often left to me to figure out how to do this. This particular brand of communist household—deeply committed to the self and to others—nurtured my three sisters and me to shoot for the moon.

My parents expected me even as a young child to know my own mind, which meant that I sometimes resisted them. They gave me the tools to chart my own course. This awareness of a self defined in and through politics allowed me to comfortably embrace feminism in my early twenties. The u.s. women's movement pushed me to look inward, from the political which was my early anchor, toward the more personal and private. With feminism, I was able to connect the objectification and exploitation of women's bodies to their own particular political exis-

tence. My female body, in and of itself, became a site to understand politically. This meant my body was also more than its individual self, and
this was newly intriguing to me.

Feminism's brilliance is found in this recognition that the body is
not simply personal, that there is a politics to sex, that personal and political life are intermeshed. This is also a dilemma for feminist theory
because more often than not personal and political, sex and power are
misinterpreted as one and the same. Instead of the same, they are similar, distinct yet also closely tied.

My feminism helped authorize my identity as something much
more than my physicality. My body is simply a part of who I am and not
my whole self. Maybe it is this feminist autonomy of the body that has
allowed me to live fully without all my body parts. My female body is
both personally political and politically personal. I live the meanings it
has absorbed from our politically charged environments, meanings I
have not completely crafted.

Breast cancer makes women fear their bodies, and hold them dear at
the same time. I have moved through much of my fear, and this opens
up new possibilities. Right now, I am not actively engaged in fighting
death, and I am sure this lets me think I have moved farther than I have.
Yet it is also true that breast cancer and death are as much a part of my
life as anything else, and that recodes all meanings. When I am feeling
brave I temper myself by actively wishing for my daughter's health.

I am trying to be open to my grief and pain so that I can enlarge it
and make it accessible to others.[2] My pain is cruelly individual but
speaks a more collective story. Disease lets us see what our lives are really made of. It is a looking glass, intensifying what matters, dismissing
what does not. Things disappear and reappear while the body heals, and
does not.

Death makes me rethink my memories and it makes new memories.
Sometimes the sadness has meant that I cannot see a future; other times
I fantasize complete control. Although the deaths of my sisters, Sarah
and Giah, splintered me with grief, they also etched new depths of lov-
ing for us. I lived their deaths with them as close to the bone as I could.
Our love felt so deep that it denied the separateness of the self. It is this

4  love that shoves me forward. Their breast cancers did not destroy our family. Instead I think we developed a new kind of communism, not in the economic sense, but in a communal sense where individual boundaries were smashed by our horrific pain.

This webbing of the personal and political is the heart of my project; and it is also its Achilles' heel. How to recombine these arenas without distorting their autonomy or dependence?

What follows is in part a political memoir, a meditation that shares the parts of my life that are something more than private reminiscences. The snapshots that follow are pieces of memory. It is hard to remember, and I know I cannot see all there is to see. I hope, however, that I can let you see how my critique of dominant breast cancer narratives stems from an unbearable, personally political pain and deep extraordinary love. By personalizing the body politic, I want to radically politicize the personal body, so that we can live differently with and against disease.

## My Family Story

If there is such a thing as genetically inherited breast cancer, I most probably have it.

My family's history of breast cancer began without any of us knowing it had started. When I first learned my beloved mother Fannie had breast cancer I had no idea what was to follow. She was forty-five years old; I was sixteen. My sisters Sarah and Giah were diagnosed while they were in their mid-twenties. My breast cancer was diagnosed when I was forty. My Aunt Nettie, my mother's sister who lived with us, was diagnosed with ovarian cancer when she was fifty-seven. I was in graduate school at the time.

I hope Julia, the youngest of us four girls, will be spared. But she has been deeply wounded by all this. Her own struggles with spinal fusion surgeries that have left her physically disabled have always existed alongside our familial crises with cancer. I fear this has left her too alone at times, because she was not dealing with death, just an unforgiving set of vertebrae. To this day she fights daily fatigue and numbing physical pain.

I play back and forth with the breast cancer master narratives that do    5
not quite fit my family's profile. Although the "self" is always a selfish
and narrowed starting point for theorizing, it is where I start, and then
move outward.

I grew up one of four daughters. Our parents were activists in the
civil rights movement. Our childhood was defined by this politics
through the late fifties and mid-sixties. The intimate love in our family
was encircled by these larger social movement commitments. There
were times I resented my parents for their political lifestyle, which just
felt too demanding to me. I disliked moving around, moving schools,
trying to make new friends, and being strong. Much of the time I just
wished I could be like other children I knew. They seemed so normal
and their lives looked so easy.

I am sure these early moments of struggle and loneliness have impacted on every part of me, including the way I have experienced breast
cancer. I know how to be alone, to be different, to try and see the larger
political corridor. So I circle outward, from my family, through our bodies, to the politics that defines them, back to the self, and outward again
to the environs we inhabit.

## My Mother Fannie

It was 1964. I had just begun college and was working hard at the
first semester of required courses. The war in vietnam defined much of
the political temper. By then the antiwar movement had begun to mobilize a serious assault against the war. Civil rights activism was still very
much on the agenda. I remember a phone message in my mailbox. I
was supposed to call home. I went to the pay phone in the lobby of my
dorm and can still see myself standing in the see-through phone booth
making the call. My father answered. His voice was tired and drawn.
Usually his energy bellowed forward. He told me that my mother had
breast cancer.

I remember being numb, not knowing how to think about this, and
then wondering, How could she have breast cancer? I just could not get
my head around the idea of this happening. The whole time I talked

6    with my dad I kept thinking that my fabulous mommy Fannie was going
to die. Looking backward, I cannot quite imagine myself then and how
unprepared I was for everything that would follow.

This was my first experience with breast cancer. Back then you
thought that breast cancer meant death . . . even if it didn't. And it did
not mean this in my mother's case. She is still alive today, at eighty-four.

At the time my mother was diagnosed, my parents and Giah and
Julia lived in Atlanta, Georgia. Sarah was in college at Radcliffe. Dad
taught at Atlanta University, the black graduate school connected to
Spelman, Clark, and Morehouse Colleges. They had been there for a
year and were already very active in the civil rights struggles for racial in-
tegration. All of them had recently been arrested while picketing Lester
Maddox's segregated restaurant. Mom had met a surgeon at several of
the demonstrations, Dr. Asa Yancey, whom she liked very much. When
she found her breast lump she called him for an appointment.

My mother's surgeon was black, and he could only practice in the
black hospital, Hughes Spalding, in Atlanta. So my mother's breast cancer operation was performed in the black hospital. My mom's radical
mastectomy for breast cancer was intimately personal and yet political.
She never considered doing anything differently than she did. This is
just who my mother is. Her life has always been devoted to civil rights. If
the hospitals were segregated, she would integrate them. The hospital
files listed her as negro; after all what else would she be? Black hospital,
black woman.

I recently contacted my mother's surgeon, Doctor Yancey, to ask
him if he remembered any racial tension at the hospital then, and he re-
sponded, no, that he did not. He did mention, however, that most of his
patients were black women owing to the laws of segregation at the time.
He himself thought nothing of the matter that my mother was white.

But I need to tell you more about my mother because she is so
much more than her, or our, cancer story. Her name is Fannie Price
Eisenstein. She was born in Rochester, New York, and her father was a
tailor and union organizer. Her mother also worked as a machine opera-
tor in the same factory as her father. They were incredibly poor through
the Depression, and she was only able to attend Cornell University

because of the full scholarship she won. The story of the scholarship exam became family folklore. While Mom was preparing for the exam there was one math problem she could not figure out. She went to all the mathematicians in Rochester until she found one who could solve the problem. And, yes, that very problem was on the exam. The political lesson in Eisenstein-communist form: there must be financial assistance so that all may have access to education, but we must also help make it happen. She went off to Cornell with a brown paper bag under her arm, which held a change of underwear.

Mom was one of the early student radicals at Cornell. Actually, according to the writer Arthur Laurents of the popular film *The Way We Were*, who also attended Cornell, Fannie Price, my mom, was a "colorful beginning for the character of [his] heroine," played by Barbra Streisand.[3] After college she worked in the Greek democratic movement during World War II, then the civil rights movement. She organized with native american women in Denver, Colorado, on land rights; assisted women on welfare in Columbus, Ohio; and led demonstrations against Woolworth's segregated lunch counters in Brooklyn, New York. Later on, after several moves around the country because my father kept losing his job, my mother became dean of adult continuing education at New York City Technical Community College, where she developed programs for black and latino women in nontraditional fields. I remember her sharing stories over dinner of programs that trained women to repair air conditioners, office machines, and the like. She raised millions in grants for these programs. My sisters and I were always intrigued with the way she would adapt her life in creative ways.

At eighty-two, she demonstrated against City University of New York's decision to limit admissions and remedial programs for primarily minority students. Her commitment to open enrollment for all students remains undiminished. She was a bit crestfallen when the police refused to put her in a paddy wagon and told her to go home at the last demonstration she participated in. She called me to complain that she was not too old to be arrested. She really is how she sounds.

She now works at the Goddard-Riverside Settlement House in Manhattan where she is involved with programs for the AIDS homeless, or-

8  ganizes against Nike and its sweatshop practices, helps people apply for what is left of welfare, and makes a difference in people's everyday lives. She is getting older but continues.

She is *also* devastated by the deaths of Sarah and Giah and Nettie. When she allows herself to weep she breaks apart. I must allow her her grief and pain, and yet I so desperately need her to protect me from it. It is unfair, but no mothers, not even my own, are allowed to crumble. We need them too much for our own strength. I now, as a mother myself, try to ease the unbearable loss for her and know I cannot.

*My Aunt Nettie*

Nettie lived with us on and off depending on where my parents' jobs took us. Whenever we found ourselves back in New York City, she would try and find an apartment big enough to hold all of us. She had a television in her bedroom and we could always sneak in and watch with her. She took each of the four of us to Europe for our first visit. She was the one who would make sure that there was some levity in our young lives. She made celebrations, in our atheist communist home, like Chanukah and Christmas, and we idolized and adored her for it.

Nettie never married and she never spoke about this unless we asked her. We did love to hear the story of how she was too poor to marry the man she loved because his parents were totally against it. It sounded like the movies. She had many wonderful women friends with whom she traveled, and she painted, and she had us. We considered her a mother along with Fannie. She truly seemed contented. She had a richly full life with no man in sight. I am sure this had a deep impact on how I thought about myself as a girl, and later as a woman. If Nettie had lived longer we would have talked much more about her life choices.

Nettie was a director of nursing for most of the years I can remember. I loved the smell of her white starched uniform and nurse's cap. We all loved to make rounds with her at her hospital. I think she played an important role in Giah and Julia's decision to do public health work. Nettie's salary was the only regular income everyone came to depend on. She was generous to all of us, and this is not a constructed false memory. Although she was less directly political than either my mother or my father, she lived as one imagines a total communist should: everything she had, from nightgowns to her little bit of savings, was for us all alike.

When Mom and Dad moved back to New York after Atlanta, they moved with Nettie to an apartment in Park Slope, Brooklyn. Giah and Julia started school, again, and it felt like maybe we would stay here for a while. Dad was directing a community center in East New York, having given up on the academy. Sarah was in graduate school at Columbia. I was the only one who had to travel home for holidays. When the building went coop Nettie decided to buy the apartment. My mother was opposed to this because she was sure they would just be forced to pull up stakes again. But Nettie was determined this time to make a home, and did. This apartment became our family place for the next thirty years. My mother has just moved from this apartment in which so much life and death took place.

Nettie had been ill for weeks with no diagnosis. She had abdominal discomfort and was having trouble breathing. For months none of the doctors at her hospital could figure out what was causing such misery. They just kept removing fluid in order to help her breathe. By the time exploratory surgery was performed her cancer had severely metastasized. We were told that she would not have more than six months to live. She began chemotherapy but it did little. I remember her death as agonizingly slow. Her devoted nursing staff cared for her round-the-clock for months. Sarah and I would sit with her and try to distract her from the pain. She died in 1971 from what I have been recently told was ovarian cancer, although I do not remember that this was the case at the time.

Nettie's death shattered my mother. Nettie was her closest friend. They were closer than blood. And this was just the beginning.

*My Sister Sarah*

Sarah was my mother's first-born. She was brilliant and somewhat shy and much less outgoing than me. Mom and Sarah shared their love

10   of literature. They both consumed books and talked about them with
immense joy. Mom loved Sarah completely and totally. One day when
my mother and I were both at the hospital with Sarah, shortly after
metastasis to the lungs was diagnosed, Mom, with tear-filled eyes, held
my hand and said: "I would give my life for her." And I simply said:
"Sarah knows." I could not swallow. I wanted to disappear. This was
such total sadness that I became someone else. My mother grieved at
Sarah's death with the same depth with which she loved her. She still
grieves, but it is more muted and silent.

Giah, younger than me in our familial lineup, was diagnosed with
her own breast cancer at the same time that Sarah was already in serious
danger. Giah was living in Michigan. She had just finished her public
health graduate degree and was working in Lansing with her first real
job. She was twenty-five.

Mom flew out to be with her for her surgery. I stayed with Sarah. I
kept wondering how Giah was coping with her own diagnosis and
Sarah's metastasis all at the same time. This was too much. I cannot really reconstruct the dizziness of this horrible time. A year later, with
Sarah struggling for her life, Giah had a second cancer in her remaining
breast. Mom went again for the surgery.

By now, Sarah had become frailer and was near death, although I remember not ever acknowledging this but knowing it. I had been traveling from Ithaca, New York, where I was teaching, to New York City as
often as I could to see her. But then Mommy Fannie called from Lansing. She said Dad had called and Sarah was failing, and that she had to
be with her. Would I come and be with Giah? I left for Lansing and
Mom left for New York.

I went to Giah and we cried for Sarah, and for Giah, and for us all.

Sarah died and my mother lost herself for a while. Looking back on
this time, I cannot recreate it. I know a part of me does not want to find
the piercing loss again. It was too complete and total. I am no longer the
same person I was when Sarah died. Neither is my mother.

I came back from Michigan and taught some classes. I was on auto-
matic pilot. I could teach but did so without really thinking. A few days
later I left Ithaca for Sarah's funeral. Her friends from Columbia and the

women's movement were all there. They spoke about her. I was numb.
Her dearest friend, Ros, reminded us all of Sarah's quiet bravery in her
fight to save her life. She also recalled for us all how Sarah fought
against the Vietnam War, and led demos for SDS (Students for a Democratic Society), and worked with MOW (Mothers on Welfare) in
Boston. I did not speak for fear of what I might say. I wanted Sarah to be
alive.

Sarah's feminism deeply defined her personhood, but I cannot really
know how this threaded into her struggles with breast cancer, or if it did.
She hated the cancer, she hated that she had lost a breast, she often told
me she would never allow herself to have a mastectomy of the other
breast. There is too much I do not know here except that our early family trials helped prepare us all for this, and it was still not enough.

Sarah and I were sixteen months apart in age. We shared a bedroom,
and sometimes we had to share a bed depending on where we were living. We shared clothes. Actually, we shared just about everything because we did not have a lot of things. I do not remember ever resenting
this, or thinking I should have more than I did, which seems strange to
me now given how much more I have and want these days.

Our parents lost too many jobs to the political intolerance of the
McCarthy times. Dad kept getting fired at one university after the next,
and Mom would take any job she could find to see us through. It
seemed cruel that the little money there was would be used for moving
costs, just to have to pick up and move again. Sometimes when Mom
and Dad were between jobs, in other words without any, we lived with
my grandfather in his tiny apartment in Brooklyn. The bed Sarah and I
slept in folded out at night. We actually thought that this was great fun
because we never liked to go to sleep anyhow. I went to bed many a
night with Sarah's flashlight on as she did her last-minute homework
scramble. Mine was usually already done.

We were sisters, and friends, especially when life seemed hard, and
it very often did. When I look back and try to reflect on these times, I
know there was distance and there were silences between us, but that is
when I look back. When we were growing up I think we thought we
were close, as people do before they deepen their ties. We depended on

12    each other and were loyal to each other's needs. I think we were happy.

When Sarah was diagnosed, I was so determined that she not feel alone—she spoke so often about how so many people just wanted to pretend that she was OK—that I spoke every thought I had to her. I wanted no silence, nothing unsaid, although I now know that there always is something left. It is after this period of being sisters—through the cancer—that I know that our early years together did not have the same depth.

Early on in our young lives we decided on our first joint political act. We sent money to the Julius and Ethel Rosenberg Defense Fund. The Rosenbergs, charged with being communist spies, had two young sons. Sarah and I were determined to help them. Although we did not have much to send—just the pennies saved through the school savings bank passbook program—we sent a combined five dollars. Sarah and I chuckled at the thought that this stupid school banking scheme, teaching us all how to be good citizens and save, allowed us to send money to help defend communist spies.

Another shared political activity was collecting for UNICEF at Halloween time. We would invariably dress up in Mom's and Aunt Nettie's clothes and say we were princesses of some sort or another. We loved putting on lipstick and painting the rest of our faces, and wearing whatever junky jewelry was lying around the house. We lived in New York City many of these years and loved its easy access Halloween night. We would canvas the big apartment buildings with focused determination. We would ring the doorbells and stick our UNICEF milk cartons out to fill while yelling "trick-or-treat for UNICEF." Nickels and pennies filled the cartons quickly. As soon as we each had our cartons full, we would run back home and then charge out again with big paper bags to get our "own" candy. Sarah always ate hers slowly and then would tease me when I had none left.

When I reflect on this time I know my memory is partial. I have vague feelings, that are almost physical, that remind me of the awkward moments of adolescence, of not really knowing oneself. Sarah and I were both kind of spindly, and silly, and just kidlike. And we also thought life was harder than we wanted it to be. We were moving a lot, had to make new friends too often, and sometimes just felt sad. We often did not know what we felt sad about but we felt it anyway.

Our parents were busy with political meetings and demos, and our home was usually filled with people. I do not remember feeling excluded or deserted, and this is probably because we were most often included in whatever was going on. When Sarah and I were old enough, we held our own placards on picket lines. For months we demonstrated every Saturday morning against Woolworth's segregated lunch counters. We chanted "Two, four, six, eight, Woolworth's should integrate," and we loved the sound of our voices. I still sometimes hear this chant in my head. We were not frightened by those who yelled back at us and told us to move to russia. We knew they were wrong.

Sarah and I used to walk to school together. We would pretend to ignore school kids who taunted us by calling us "commies." Sarah would tell them to shut up. I loved it when she acted like my big sister even though as we got older I became the more combative one. She had a calm restraint about her while I developed a big mouth.

When the family moved from New York City to Columbus, Ohio, Sarah stayed in New York with Aunt Nettie and Grandpa for her senior year of high school. Dad had gotten a job at Ohio State University. I would begin high school by myself, without Sarah. In Ohio I was singled out in my high school not only as the daughter of communists, but as the only jew. To this day I wonder how these rumors start. After all, we were atheist. How did they even know I was a jew? I had really gotten tired of all the strife and I missed Sarah horribly. I started just wanting to fit in, and did not, and didn't have Sarah. Giah was still too young to give me much comfort, and so was Julia. I really began to wish that my parents were different—more like everyone else.

I started working hard at fitting in, which was easier than I had imagined. I did not reject my parent's values, but I just decided to keep my thoughts to myself at school. I made friends and I was having fun. Meanwhile, Sarah went off to Radcliffe for college the next year and became very politically involved with SDS. She had at first thought she would become a doctor, but quickly changed her mind. She switched majors and took classes in the social relations department with Barrington

14 Moore. My father was not pleased. This switch was too close to the choices made in his own life.

Sarah had also fallen in love and began living with Hal. She called from Cambridge to tell my parents of this, and that she was going to start taking birth control pills. We were pretty open in my family, and I guess in part this was because the zone of privacy was less given our parents' political views. Our personal lives were not completely our own to decide, just as any money we earned went into the family pot. I remember my father blowing up at Sarah and trembling with anger through the phone.

Dad yelled at Sarah with total disgust. He completely condemned her choice of taking the pill. He did not think the pill was a good idea because so little was known about its effects. I'm sure my father's upset was a personal/political mix of his disdain for a science dependent on the profit motive *and* a father's patriarchal protection of his daughter's sexuality. But he could not forbid her, and this was also who he was; this was her personal choice. When Sarah died, Dad could not forgive himself for allowing her to take the pill. But, of course, this is the awful pain of death that pushes you to think you could have made a difference. Sarah would have taken the pill no matter what Dad said.

My father lost his job in Columbus just as he thought he would be granted tenure, and we moved to Atlanta, Georgia, for my senior year of high school. This was the first time I noticed how hard the constant moving was for my mother. She had a settlement house job she loved on the South Side in Columbus, organizing women on welfare. She did not want to move. I wanted to remain in Ohio but for far different reasons. I had become mainstream and I liked it. But my parents thought I had become too at ease with being one of the crowd. I had to move to Atlanta for my senior year.

It was a horrible year. I could barely stand my own anger and the tension of it. Schools, then, were still racially segregated. We lived in black Atlanta and I attended an all-white high school. I still was the girl who had walked the picket lines, but I was also not strong enough to sort out how I could bridge the gulfs that divided me. I cannot, or won't,

reconstruct the sadness of my life then. My parents and Giah and Julia    15
were always demonstrating and being arrested. I was not. In that year, I
hated my parents and felt enormously alone.

Meanwhile, Sarah was thriving and actively engaged with the student movement. We drifted apart while she was at Radcliffe, and more
so when I went back to Ohio for college. When we each entered graduate school we started moving back toward each other. She was active in
the Columbia student movement and was arrested in the student upris-
ing demanding that the university be more responsible to its surrounding neighborhoods. I was home at the time—which was back in New
York—on break from graduate school when my parents got the call to
make bond and went and got her. I was surprised at how unsettled Dad
seemed. This New Left politics was not his kind.

After several years of sorting out the different parts of myself, I finally
felt I had figured out my own brand of political self. I then became active in the women's movement while in grad school. My blending of
feminism and socialism was also hard for my dad, even though he was
the one to teach me always to think things through for myself, to the
core. Mom was more open. By this time Sarah was also involved in the
SDS part of feminism. We each had found our own way through to our
personal politics.

We went together to the first Women's March to the Pentagon,
against the Vietnam War in 1971. She spoke at the rally on behalf of the
women factory workers she was writing her dissertation about: the girls
and women who had died in the early 1900s in the Triangle Shirtwaist
factory fire. She spoke of them and the women of vietnam as one.

Sarah's life was full and determined, but then cancer interfered with
this. She was diagnosed with stage-one breast cancer while writing her
dissertation, "Bread and Roses." (Hal saw that this was published a few
years after Sarah died.)

I need to back up here. Sarah called me in Ithaca, New York, where
I now lived, to tell me she had found a lump in her breast. She had already been to the doctor, who had said it was probably nothing to worry
about given she was just twenty-something. He had suggested a biopsy

16  and removal of the lump. She was going into the hospital the next day for the procedure, and she wanted me to know. I said I would come to be with her. She said it was not necessary, that it was nothing.

The next day came, and Mom called me, instead of Sarah. The lump had been removed but it was not nothing, it was malignant. Sarah would need to have a mastectomy. She had not been asked to sign papers agreeing to a mastectomy if necessary, which was protocol at the time, because her surgeon was sure it was nonmalignant. I know today that a two-stage procedure is the one of choice. But back then, I kept thinking of Sarah in her hospital bed, waiting all over again for the next procedure. I wanted all this to go away, and it would not. She had the mastectomy.

From the start, I never thought Sarah would die. I had thought my mom was going to die when I learned that she had breast cancer, but that was a long time ago and Mom was still OK, and so I thought Sarah would be too. Although I ached for Sarah, and worried about how she felt about her new body, I thought she would live. I realize now that I just assumed all the breast cancer had been removed, because no nodes were involved and the doctor said she should be fine.

I traveled into the city and helped Sarah walk the walls with her arm to stretch the scar tissue. At the time she was diagnosed there was no talk of chemotherapy treatments for any possible renegade cells left. So there was little else medically to do. We all went on with our lives. Sarah just no longer had one of her breasts. Neither did Mom. Life could still be wonderful.

The next three years were pretty much like any other set of three. At the time I did not know I would never live life that way again, as a person who assumes that life just goes on. But only three years after surgery, Sarah developed a soreness on her chest bone that was worrisome. She did not tell me or Mom or Dad and instead went with Hal to see her surgeon, who opted for exploratory surgery. The breast cancer had metastasized to her lung. Sarah had lung cancer.

It was very early morning when the phone rang. It was Dad, and I knew that his voice was not his own. I knew deep within me that something was very wrong. He cried first and then he spoke. He told me that the cancer had spread to Sarah's lung. For the first time since all this began I thought that Sarah was going to die. *My beloved Sarah is going to die.* I left for New York City to be with her. I dreaded knowing I would have to look her in the eyes. On the plane down, I made myself practice looking straight at her. What would be my first words? "I'm sorry" would not do. These words did not even begin to say anything. She demanded honesty and closeness from me but I did not think I could do this. I did not even know what honesty meant here.

Over the next two years we rode the cancer roller coaster of hope and despair. At times I made myself believe that Sarah could will herself to live. I made more and more time to be with her even though I was living in Ithaca.

Her chemotherapy treatments drained her of her energy. She lost her hair except for a few determined wisps that refused to fall out. I went with her to get a wig, but she did not like the feel of it. Instead we bought the most beautiful head scarves we could find. I did not know which was harder for her body to sustain, the cancer or the chemo, and I also knew it did not matter which it was. I found all the yogurt recipes I could to help keep her yeast balance normal. I would sit in her living room and quietly keep her company. I would help her slowly move to the bathroom. I can still feel myself sitting in her living room.

Sarah loved to cook and she was totally gourmet. But she was not cooking now. She was still determined to create a gourmet luncheon for me to celebrate publication of my first book. So from her couch she instructed Hal on all her favorite food stores and asked him to bring back every kind of delicacy imaginable. Even though she was beyond eating much, and in considerable pain, she sat at the table and toasted the first edition of *Capitalist Patriarchy and the Case for Socialist Feminism* with a house filled with wonderful friends. I still feel the glow of her love as she held up her glass and looked my way. I was forcing myself to celebrate and grieve at the same time. If Sarah could do this, I must. On that particular day I thought miraculous Sarah could not die.

Sarah hated the cancer. She hated the way people who were healthy acted as if their health were a sign of their goodness. She hated the pretense of people who could not deal with her cancer. She would tell me

18  how she would walk down the street and just want to give her cancer away to someone else. She told me often how she did not want to die. I still hear her.

Hal and Sarah lived together for almost twenty years. After her metastasis they decided to marry. Sarah had always thought marriage was unnecessary, but now, if she died, she wanted a record that she and Hal had been together. Being Sarah, she also just wanted to have a huge party, in defiance of it all. We all made a fabulous celebration, and I had to grieve and celebrate at the same time again. Mom and Dad did the cooking and it was glorious. I was in charge of the flowers. Sarah's favorites were irises, so the house was filled with them. Friends from everywhere came. On this day too I thought it was impossible that she could die.

Sarah started having dizzy spells. She started losing her balance and falling. The dizziness became more regular. Tests showed that the cancer had spread to her brain. Her beautiful bald head now had markings for the radiation sites. No part of her body was the same, except, as she joked, her feet. I began to see an end coming. I kept trying not to be sad or scared, and then it would be as if she were not dying.

I now knew that Sarah was dying, although it is impossible to say what this really means. Death is so final and complete, you cannot really know it until it comes, and then it is over and becomes something else. I did know, however, that I would savor every moment. I would love her every possible way so that she would have to know how much I loved her. I would make myself remember this love for the rest of my life. When I can bear it, I allow myself to live with these memories for days, and then I say good-bye until I find myself grieving again.

In the last few weeks of her life Sarah rested in her living room. She was quieter. We would talk softly, and sometimes not at all. Sometimes she would say that she did not want someone else to be with Hal after her. She would lose full consciousness and speak of Mom and how she wished she could spare her. I did not want to be far from that room. I felt close to her there, and less lonely.

Sarah reentered the hospital after I left for Ithaca. She died a few days later. On that day, Mom had already left for the hospital. My father was still at home and took the call from the nurse. Sarah had died and Mom was already on her way to see her. My mother would enter Sarah's room and she would already be dead. The oxygen would be unhooked and there would just be white sheets. My father called me to tell me that Mom was riding the subway and did not even know. He just kept repeating himself. My father died just a year after Sarah. He had a massive heart attack at age sixty-one. In part his heart had been broken by the loss of his first-born; but it had already been severely wounded through an earlier heart attack during his years of political battle. His death has always felt very politically personal to me.

I got off the phone and called my friends Miriam and Isaac to take me to the airport. Then I called Giah to tell her Sarah had died. Giah, still weak from her own surgery, could never forgive that she was unable to say good-bye to Sarah. I was never lonelier than I was on that plane ride. Julia was already on her way to New York.

## My Sister Giah

Giah was four years younger than me. My sisters used to tease me that my parents were eager to have another child after Sarah—hence the closeness of our ages—but after me they waited for another four years.

Giah was energetic and moody, extremely vivacious and somewhat volatile. She was athletic with a strong body and big breasts. She loved to swim and to folk dance. We did not share the women's movement as Sarah and I did, but we shared being sisters. She was very loving and generous to me.

Life in Atlanta was especially hard for Giah and Julia. I lived there only for my senior year of high school, made life difficult for everyone in the family that year, and then left for college. But Giah and Julia lived there for another three complicated years, and they were younger. Many of the children at the grammar school they attended were openly racist. They threatened and bullied my younger sisters. They taunted Giah and Julia for having a father who taught at the "nigger school" and for living in the "nigger neighborhood." At one point my parents had to

20   have them escorted to and from school to protect them. Giah was pretty fearless through this period and protected Julia, who was just too young for some of this brutality.

Giah's defiant personality was already evident at age eleven. She had been picketing with Mom, Dad, and Julia. They were arrested, and Giah and Julia were separated from my parents and put in a different paddy wagon. When Giah insisted that she would not leave Julia, who was eight years old at the time, the warden at the juvenile detention center put Giah on bread and water and told her to shut up. Later, when the water came, Giah refused to drink it on command. I found Giah completely confident when civil rights activist and professor Staughton Lynd and I went to bring them home.

Mom and Dad remained in jail for several days. Mom was put in solitary confinement. Dad was lucky enough to share a cell with comedian Dick Gregory. Several weeks later a young black civil rights lawyer whose name I cannot retrieve from my memory defended my parents against charges of parental delinquency—for allowing such young children to be on a picket line. He won.

Giah was too young, like Sarah, when she was diagnosed with her breast cancers. She was just starting her first real job post–grad school, and Sarah was already dealing with metastasis. Giah went through her surgeries while we all tried to be attentive to her and Sarah. She had to share us when she deserved total devotion. I still cannot imagine her agony as she struggled past her mastectomies while Sarah was dying.

Giah knew how sad I was. She knew how deeply I loved Sarah. I learned from Giah that she too wanted extraordinary love from me. Before Giah died, I did love her this way. Giah also knew how much I wanted her to be brave, to work at getting strong, and to live. I spent time in Lansing, helping Giah walk the walls with each of her arms. I tried to comfort her as she mourned the loss of her voluptuous breasts. I kept telling her how beautiful she still was, but she could not hear me. Time passed, and Giah healed some.

In a few years, Giah married Jim, a canadian attorney. She was feeling pressure to change her name and asked me if I could forgive her if she did. I told her I would never speak to her again if she did so, so she stayed Eisenstein. She moved to Toronto to be with Jim and took a job with the Ministry of Health. She was incredibly effective at her job and even succeeded in bringing down the barbed wire fencing that had encircled minimum security mental health facilities. She was really proud to have done this. She also birthed two children, Jeremy and Corenne.

Several years passed and Giah decided she wanted another child. I was completely set against this. She had just finally gotten on top of her job and the tough early years of childhood. Another child was too much. I worried for her health. It would be too much stress. I was furious that she made me ask: "What if the cancer returns?" And she answered as she always had: "It won't." I had deeply admired her full embrace of life when she decided on having Jeremy and Corenne, but not this time. What if she were to die? How would Jim manage? She did not listen. Giah was determined to live her life without fear. Instead of one more child, twins were born, Devon and Kyle.

Jim's law firm was moving to Calgary. I selfishly asked Giah not to go. I knew that it was too far away for me to be helpful to her if she got sick again. I said that Jim should look for something else, that her work at the Ministry was too important to leave. She said she was ready for a job change anyway. I once again brought up the possibility of her having a recurrence. Giah said she would be all right. I was really worried for Giah, but decided to follow her lead. Pretty soon they all moved. I kept thinking Calgary was too far away.

Four years later Giah started not to feel well. She was overly tired and had some abdominal discomfort. She saw her doctors, who first diagnosed her as depressed and/or suffering from bad PMS. After a while she was diagnosed with a nervous bowel. After several more months Giah was really worried. She knew something was wrong. I keep wondering if all this might have been different if she had stayed in Toronto with the doctors who really knew her. But of course this changes nothing now.

I will never quite forget the evening she called me crying. She was distraught. She said she felt constant pressure in her abdomen and that

22    she was swollen as though she were pregnant. She never mentioned the
      word cancer. I remember my heart stopping. I had read quite a bit about
      these symptoms. I thought, my god, Giah has ovarian cancer.

          I tried to calm my fear and rage. I told her she must see a gynecolog-
      ical oncologist immediately, and that I worried she had ovarian cancer. I
      hated myself. She hung up the phone and I knew this was a terrible new
      beginning. The CA125 test was done for ovarian cancer, but it came
      back negative, as it often will. Her condition worsened. In the next days
      liquid was drained from her abdomen. Cancer cells were now depicted
      in the liquid. By the time she was operated on her cancer had spread;
      only a partial hysterectomy could be performed given the extent of
      metastasis. She was at stage-four ovarian cancer.

          I had been here before. I thought, I am going to lose Giah too. But I
      forced myself from these thoughts.

          After the surgery she underwent a grueling regime of chemotherapy
      that shrank much of the cancer that they could not remove. Was this a
      reprieve? We hoped against hope. A second surgery was performed to
      see if the shrinkage would allow further removal of the tumor. Some fur-
      ther removal of the cancer was possible. It looked like Giah had a fight-
      ing chance. She underwent two more abdominal surgeries along with
      more chemo treatments. Her protocol was unrelenting and horrendous
      but she fought like an animal. She was determined to stay alive and
      would force herself to do so. I walked around with a constant aching.
      Her twins were just six years old.

          The news was good. Tests showed there was a major remission.
      Could she have beaten stage-four ovarian? If anyone could, Giah could.

          Within two months we were grieving again. Cancer cells had reap-
      peared. I knew that the only chance Giah had of surviving would be a
      bone marrow transplant. I needed to talk with her and her doctors.
      Maybe her doctors thought she would not agree and therefore had not
      suggested the transplant. I did not know or care. I just wanted Giah to
      take this last chance.

          It was torture to make the call. I called Giah and asked that she con-
      sider doing a bone marrow transplant. She said she couldn't. I said it was

her only chance; that without it she would die. She was silent at the other end. We had not talked about dying. She was different from Sarah this way. She never mentioned dying. It was out of the question.

She said she was terrified of the T-cell removal and the horrific side effects. I said I was too, and that I would come, and that I would stay in the hospital with her through the first treatment. That I would not leave her side and that she would survive it. She said she had to think about it. We hung up. I cried but it changed nothing. I missed my sister Sarah. It was lonelier without her. I wanted Giah to live. Meanwhile Julia was having to consider yet one more spinal fusion surgery.

I traveled to Calgary the next week to be with Giah for the transplant. This time when I left Ithaca I was leaving behind my ten-year-old daughter, Sarah, named after my sister, and her father, Richard. My daughter was so reluctant to let me go, believing that I was OK only if she could see me. She loved her Aunt Giah and did not want her to die like Aunt Sarah.

I went straight to Foothills Hospital from the airport. Unit 5A was for transplant patients. I had to disinfect myself and take careful precautions before entering the ward or Giah's room. I felt strange wondering for a split second if I might be on a ward like this myself someday. But that was not important at this particular moment as I entered Giah's room.

Giah had shaved her head and looked quite stunning despite the horror of it all. They had started the drugs earlier in the day. But I was grateful to have arrived to help her through the vomiting. Her mouth had horrible sores. Her body shook uncontrollably until I got on the bed and held her so tight that she could not move. I iced the parts of her body that were tender. The episodes are indescribable, and they took Giah and me to someplace else together.

As soon as there was a lull, and Giah regrouped, we would walk through the halls of the ward and laugh together. These were incredible moments. There was nothing to come between us, or divert us. We were just there together fighting for her to stay alive. Then we would wait for the next episode and ride it through.

24    I returned home. There were two more treatments that beloved friends and Mom came for. Then the treatments ended. All there was to do now was wait and see.

Just two months later, before any of us were ready to hear such news, her blood work showed a recurrence. I did not want to believe the report. How could this be, and so soon? The transplant had done nothing.

I knew we were approaching an end and could not face it. Giah would acknowledge no such thing. She started a different treatment regime of Taxol. She became frailer and weaker and needed a wheelchair to get around. Her voice became fainter over the phone so that I could barely hear her. Mom was in and out of Calgary and saw Giah wasting away. Giah became a ghost of herself. Then Mom could not leave her. She knew Giah would be gone soon.

I got a ticket to return to Calgary in a few days. I had to try and prepare my daughter Sarah before I left. Giah's struggle had been deeply wounding to Sarah and she was fearful for me. Sarah kept asking me not to be so sad. I knew what Sarah needed from me because I have needed the same from my own mother. I needed to make sure she was all right before I left in case I would be gone for a while.

Mom was not sure Giah would live long enough to see me. At this point I did not think I could bear to see Giah alive and dying. So I waited the few days to go, but so did Giah.

I once again entered Foothills Hospital. I took the elevator to the third floor. It was already 11:00 P.M. My plane was late. But, actually, time had already stopped for me. I could hardly navigate through my tears and terror as I walked toward her room. Her door was almost closed. A sign read: DO NOT ENTER WITHOUT SPEAKING TO A NURSE. I knew the sign was not meant for me; her sister who loved her and already knew. The sign meant that Giah was past consciousness.

I entered her room and forced myself not to see her emaciated body and instead to remember my gorgeous, noisy, brave younger sister. When I bent over to hold what was left of Giah she slowly lifted her arms and embraced me. No words came forth from her. She had been lying silent and still for days. Giah's brief embrace of my body touched straight through to my soul. I still can feel her touch.

I sat beside her for the next hours and held her hand. Her face and body looked like a Holocaust victim's. I just sat there and could not be anywhere else. Night came and I went to her home to try and sleep a bit. Mom stayed, sitting in a chair at the base of her bed. I can still see her.

I could not sleep, so the phone call from my mother, before dawn, did not wake me. Mom just said my name. There were no words left to say.

I got dressed and went to the hospital. I cried with the nurses but we said nothing. Her children went into the room where Giah still lay, and horrible sounds of pain and sorrow came through the walls. I thought I had no tears left, but they came.

Giah's body was removed. I kept touching my mother to let her know she was not alone.

That night I put Giah's twins to bed. I do not know how I did this. I tried to read them a story when Kyle asked me why his mommy had to die. I talked for what seemed like forever, trying to lovingly explain the unexplainable, and said everything I could think of to help him through his untouchable sadness. "People die, and there is no reason. Death comes and it must be taken as part of how we live." He listened and cried while I spoke and then still asked: "But why my mommy?" I sobbed with him and just held him tight.

Giah will be dead four years this month. I still see her in my closet where clothes she has given me hang. I think of her each time I move the candlesticks on my dining room table that she sent when she was already too sick to do so. I still sometimes think it is impossible that Giah fought against her breast cancers only in the end to be brutalized by ovarian cancer. I force myself to remember all else that she was. Sometimes I can. Sometimes I cannot. I revisit the pain and loss to make sure she remains a part of me, and I repress it when I can't stand it. But I never know when a visit is coming.

My doctors pushed me to have my ovaries removed as soon as Giah was diagnosed. I did so, first chance I had, so that I would recover and be able to travel to see Giah. Meanwhile, every other part of one's life still moves forward. This surgery, so close to Giah's diagnosis, was hard

26    for my daughter Sarah. She did not want to hear about one more hospital stay. She did not want to hear that I needed to have my body carved in order to protect it.

On my bad days I feel castrated and amputated. On my good days I do not care. It is just sometimes hard to live knowing that Giah may have saved my life.

## My Own Cancer

I was taking a shower. It felt like a hard pea. I called my gynecologist and made an appointment to see her. I had my period and hoped that the lump would disappear. We were going on vacation, so we left. Each day I would check to see if the hard lump was still there, and it was. I probably was checking myself hourly. Rich kept asking if I still felt it. I kept hoping.

I had become practiced at splitting myself. I knew how to have fun and still be worried at the same time. We hiked and biked and played with our daughter, Sarah, who was three at the time. A three year old can almost push all else to the side.

When we got back home I kept my appointment. Katherine, my gynecologist, did not think the lump felt suspicious, that it was more cyst-like, but given my family history she wanted a surgeon to check it out immediately. She made some calls. Three days later I was sitting in Rob MacKenzie's surgical suite of offices. I remember trying to make myself not think. I suspended thought and feelings too. I don't think I thought about anything while I sat there.

The nurse called my name. I walked into the room and met with MacKenzie. He felt the hardness and did not think it was a liquid cyst. If this was so, it would not aspirate. There was no way really to know anything without a biopsy. Usually he would wait and see but he thought we should not wait in my case. I will always cherish his concern for me that day.

It was already late in the afternoon. He asked if I could cope with a biopsy on the spot if one of his nurses was willing to stay past five. I said of course I could.

They prepped me and I was still not thinking. I was saving my energy and my thoughts. Living with cancer has taught me an incredible discipline. I try not to throw away my energy on worry and sadness in advance of knowing. MacKenzie removed the tumor and showed it to me. He thought it looked benign, but could not really tell until the tests were run. I went home and took some Tylenol to ease the slight discomfort in my breast. I was on hold.

The phone rang on the early side, Saturday morning. It was Rob MacKenzie. His voice told me everything I needed to know without his saying anything more. I knew and didn't. He told me he was sorry. After all these years I too had breast cancer. No tears. No why me. Just . . . nothing. "No, I did not need to see him right then. . . . I was OK . . . just needed some time . . . I would see him Monday."

My mind was short-circuiting. Rich was downstairs with Sarah. I had to tell Rich. I thought, I cannot tell my mother, or Julia. . . this is just too cruel. And what of little Sarah? She will be so frightened. I just wanted to be quiet.

It was stage one. Protocol by this time usually meant lumpectomy for most women with follow-up radiation and chemotherapy. The chemos were pretty mild by now—little or no hair loss, vague nausea. Or there was tamoxifen if you were estrogen receptor sensitive.

MacKenzie thought that mastectomy was probably the appropriate option for me. Given my family's track record, why chance another tumor? Why use my energy wondering about another cancer? This felt right.

My oncologist agreed, but thought about my options differently. She thought I should have the mastectomy for cosmetic reasons. She thought my breast would look better after mastectomy and reconstruction than after a lumpectomy.

I wondered why she was so much more focused on the cosmetics than on the recurrence of cancer for me. Statistical guides are one thing, and my individual familial predisposition quite another. Either way, mastectomy was advised, but I was not sure I liked how she thought things through. I actually wasn't sure I liked her at all.

On the other hand, because of my family history, she recommended

28  that I undergo a radical chemo protocol using adryamycin. She thought this would give me my best shot at not having a recurrence, even though the drug was difficult to sustain. Yes, my hair would fall out and I would be quite sick from the treatment. She said she could give me drugs for the nausea but they would knock me out. I decided on low-level anti-nausea drugs so that I could retain a part of myself through this.

I decided on mastectomy so that I would not feel hostage to my breast. But I did not know what to do about chemo. I only had stage one, and little was known about long-term effects of adryamycin. But my sister Sarah had also been stage one and died. I was desperate not to do the adryamycin. I hated the thought of vomiting my way through thirty-six hours of hell. I hated the thought of losing my fabulous hair. I hated the idea of deep fatigue. I hated all of this. I was racked with uncertainty because I so wanted to live and watch my daughter grow.

I lost ten pounds from the nausea of just thinking about whether to do the chemo. Everyone who loves me loved me too much to ask me to do the chemo. They felt they could not pressure me. In the end, on the night I had been given as a deadline to decide, my mother called and hesitantly and softly said to me, "There wasn't chemo for Sarah, and Giah did it preventively and is still fine." That is all she could say. She had lived through Sarah's chemo treatments after her metastasis and could not ask me to do this to myself. I hung up the phone, and Rich, his voice filled with tears, said, "Zillah, please." So I did.

I had my mastectomy and found it much less difficult than I had imagined. I did not think about my breast. It was gone. The love that surrounded me shielded me from a sense of loss. There was just too much to be thankful for. I was looking in this direction and not to my chest.

Maybe I had said good-bye to my breast long before it was taken from me. I do not really know. I just know I have a different body now. I like my body. I would never have chosen any of this, but what does that really mean? This is what life is.

I am sure that my memories of this period are partial. I can still feel the process of pulling at my brain, ordering it to not wander, and just to do what I needed from it at the moment. I had little pain after the surgery. It was nothing compared with the postpartum agony of child-birth. When my surgeon removed the early set of bandages, I mumbled to myself: "This doesn't look so bad." That was a first for him.

The aftereffects of the anesthesia were a different story. I vomited and was dizzy for days. I wanted to throw the Reach for Recovery women out of my room but just asked them to leave. I did not want to hear or listen to them feel sorry for me. I did not need their pieces of white gauze for my chest. I would leave the hospital my own way.

Little Sarah and Rich came to the hospital the evening of surgery and I swallowed my nausea. I could do just about anything to protect Sarah from seeing my weakened state. We ate chinese food on my hospital bed and she chatted away as if nothing was strange, except she would not let go of my hand. We each ate one-handed. Every cell in my body was determined that I live to see this sweet child of mine grow.

Chemotherapy started a few weeks later. I never rethought the decision. I just went forward. Beginning several hours after each of the six treatments, I would vomit violently for fourteen hours. I threw-up every thirty-two minutes as a wild wave of nausea rippled through me, and then crested. For these hours life was little else but the chemo. Three to four days of deadening nausea would follow, but the nausea just was there, it did not keep me from my life.

I felt triumphant getting through the chemo. I kept teaching and chaired the department of politics, ran four miles every day except the two days after treatment with my friends Carla and Patty who said we can always walk. During the six-month siege we even went on a pro-abortion march to Washington, D.C. Miriam, Isaac, and Rich took turns helping me and pushing Sarah's carriage. I so much wanted Sarah to know that there is always a bigger political picture that we fit into. I was on chemo, but I would not allow it to smash everything else.

Richard stayed within arm's reach for the fourteen-hour posttreatment ordeal. Students adjusted their schedules to mine. Miriam drove me to each treatment and talked nonstop as the red liquid dripped into my veins. My daughter's day-care teachers, Rosie and Diane, always spent the night of chemo with us in our home. Dear lifelong friends Ellen or Ros, or beloved Mommy Fannie came to stay at my home on

30    the weekend following the treatments to cook, and play with Sarah, and remind me of their love. Friends in town brought food. The staffs at my doctor's offices became friends. I did not do chemo alone.

Rich, Sarah, and I went to Sanibel Island to celebrate the end of the red stuff but it was too early for me to celebrate. Although I loved watching Sarah play in the waves, and trundle down the beach with her juice bottle hanging from her mouth with no hands, I was grieving inside. Everyone looked so healthy here. No one else had breast cancer, I was sure. When I would walk along the beach by myself, my almost bald head was read as "dyke." Normally, that would have been fine, but not now, not when it made the pain in my life invisible. Strange world.

After a four-month rest from the adryamycin, I had prophylactic surgery on my right breast. Giah's second breast cancer weighed heavily in this decision. My cancer was lobular, which often means it will occur bilaterally. I did not want to risk another round of chemo down the road. Rob MacKenzie, at my request, did this surgery using local anesthetic. The first time around, the general anesthesia had been worse than the operation for me. When I asked him to use local this time, he hesitated and said he needed to think about it. I told him I could handle it. The anesthesiologist told me I was making a big mistake and the nurses wished I would not do this.

The surgery seemed to take forever. I felt no pain, but a disconcerting pressure in my chest that I still sometimes return to when I daydream. I'm not sure I could do it again, but I will never have to know. The recovery was completely simple—no nodes are removed when it's a healthy breast so it is less intrusive. And the local anesthesia wore off quickly. I was able to go running two days later but maybe pushed too much. I developed a postoperative embolism where my breast had been. I was once again on the operating table with Rob standing over me. I had to promise MacKenzie I would not run for ten days. I kept my promise.

I spoke with Rob recently, wondering whether he has changed over time as a breast cancer surgeon. Protocols have changed and today most of the surgeries he does are lumpectomies. He says that he, as well as his patients, has become more open in dealing with breast cancer. When I asked him if mastectomies or lumpectomies were harder for him to do than other surgeries, given our breast culture, he said no, that cutting the face was the hardest for him. I never ask myself today whether I should have just done lumpectomies. It is an impossible question.

By now, two of my dearest friends, Miriam and Ellen, who shared in each step of my particular protocol, have dealt with their own breast cancers. They had lumpectomies and follow-up radiation. Miriam did a low-dose chemo, and Ellen is on tamoxifen. We have shared each of these decisions deeply and profoundly because the decisions are complex and individually personal.

Thinking backward to the difficult period of chemo I see my wild red wigs. One had a million curls, the other was a straight banged page-boy. Neither was anything like my real hair. Just because I had no choice about getting breast cancer did not mean that I was going to live it passively. I would finally have the hair I had fantasized at age sixteen. I flew down to New York and got my wigs. I did not try to look the same as before, and did not. I mapped my own cancer look. I would switch wigs depending on my mood, and people would get confused and wonder how my hair could look so different one day to the next. I would think: You must be kidding. These are wigs. I am on chemo. You must know that. How can you not know this? I would tell them and they would not hear.

I am vain, and losing my hair was horrible. I remember the night that most of my hair simply fell out when I tried to comb it. I can still see the trash can in the bathroom filled with me. But I just see it and cannot touch how I felt then. Sarah would demand to wear the wigs around the house, but afterward she never wanted to see them again.

The horror of chemo freed a part of me. I became more convinced than ever that women let others regulate and discipline our bodies too much, and that we can take more control. That goes for our doctors and the people we think are watching us. People do not really notice or see as much as we see ourselves. I was so tense to walk out into the world in my wigs, and most of the world did not even notice. A colleague at school said, "Something is different, what's different?" I try to act as though my body is my own to craft however I wish.

32   But this is not simply true. When I am showering after African dance class, or aerobics, or a run, I hang my towel over my chest so that women in the gym will not see my chest if they do not want to. When I am meeting people for the first time, I usually wear my prostheses, while I seldom do at home with friends. I wear prostheses less frequently, but I still wear them when I do not want to negotiate the world through my breast cancer.

In the beginning, Sarah needed me to have breasts, so I wore specially filled bras I had made for me. I wouldn't wear the traditional prostheses because they sat too awkwardly on my chest wall of muscle. The forms were too big. The mastectomy bras were too ugly and matronly. I bought the prettiest bras I could find in small sizes and had them filled with cotton. They were light and easy. I kept lifting weights and developing my own cleavage.

Before my mastectomies I hardly ever wore a bra.

I have and have had several bodies. My needs have shifted and changed over the last ten years. When I go running I now usually run with my chest free. I have learned to live with my body in new ways. Sarah has been a part of this process because her needs are also my own. She has become much freer about my surgeries, and so have I. But the freedom is still delineated within a masculinist breast-conscious world which itself constructs the meanings of breast cancer. So I am not completely free and I am also defiant. I wear my prostheses as I wear my jewelry and clothes; often as costume.

I wish I could talk to Audre Lorde about this now. She was a black lesbian feminist who after her mastectomy in 1978 bravely rejected wearing a prosthesis and wrote about it in *The Cancer Journals*.[4] She thought wearing a prosthesis was a form of lying, of covering up the trauma of breast cancer. She chose to be a militant one-breasted woman rather than practice what she felt was deceit. She asserted her one breastedness in order to make breast cancer visible. Lumpectomy has of course changed the issue of (in)visibility. As well, I wonder whether I want breast cancer to be a visible identity, and what that means for an individual.

It is many years later and I am not sure there is one truth or form of militancy today. There is no one breast cancer identity for me because it

changes along with the rest of me. It is a disease I never want to be    33
wholly defined by. I negotiate its meaning and its place in my life over
and over again. I have reconstructed my own body while my body is
never wholly mine to define. I have chosen my flesh over silicon or
saline, but sometimes this is not enough. So I clearly do not want a
breast cancer identity plastered onto me.

A somewhat enlarged node developed under my left arm, the side of
my first mastectomy, around the five-year mark, but it passed. Close to
my ten-year anniversary, blood tracing showed my sugar level was up. Is
my pancreas in trouble? Another test showed the sugar as OK. Some
days my stomach is bloated and I feel tired and I wonder; and then I
don't. My lower back is starting to give me trouble. I think this is *not*
cancer. But who knows. I get a new pair of running shoes to cushion me
more. I both completely know my body and fear it too. It is twelve years
this month.

## My Daughter Sarah

My daughter Sarah is now fifteen. She has a wondrous youthful
body that is blossoming. I have to make sure to help her through this
time when her body is beginning to look so different from mine. In a
family like ours there is much to fear, and I do not want her fearful. I
usually talk more than she does about all this. She often tries to hush me
by saying, "I know, Mom." When I ask her how she feels as my daughter
about my body, she promises that she loves my body the way it is, that
she does not really remember my breasts anymore. I know she is not vis-
iting all her feelings, although she has recently begun to open some new
doors. I so deeply want to give her the space she needs to be who she
needs to be. Bra shopping with me cannot be simple for her.

Telling Sarah I was going into the hospital to have a mastectomy, to
have my breast removed, was so complicated for me. I was incredibly
sad and did not want to share this with her, but also knew how well she
knows me. Yet I did not know what she would be able to understand.
She was extremely verbal at three, but that did not seem to help me to
know how to tell her. She cried bitterly, mainly about my going to a

34    hospital and being away from her for several days. She was inconsolable.
I do not know what she thought about the mastectomy itself. For the
next days we read a children's book about going to the hospital over and
over and over again.

Sarah, to this day, swears that we never told her the truth about the
mastectomy. She says that we told her that my breast had gotten caught
in a car door. I have no idea from where this story derives. Somehow,
she finds the story comforting. She knows who she is named after.

When I first came home from the hospital after my surgery Sarah
seemed a bit frightened around me. She held back and would watch me
from a distance. We had always been very physical with each other so I
was keenly aware of her change. I knew I had to help her and I also
wanted to give her the distance she needed. As soon as my wound had
healed enough for me to bathe, I asked her to take a bath with me. Our
daily baths together had been a very special relaxing time when we
would play and be close. I actually think it was her favorite daily routine
with me. But now she just shook her head no and scurried away. I
thought as deeply as I could, and wondered whether she could not look
at my scar, whether she did not want to see what had been done to my
chest. I walked over to her, took her in my arms, and said, "I will wear a
T-shirt, will that make it better?" A big smile crossed her face and we
headed toward the tub.

I wore the shirt for her for the next month. I chose not to say anything more until she was ready. I knew that she could not say what she
needed to say to me, that she would be too fearful of hurting me. Then
one day, with one leg already in the bath, Sarah said, "Mommy, you
don't need to wear it anymore." I asked her if she were sure and told her
that I really did not mind wearing a shirt. She nodded her head yes, she
was really sure. I took off my shirt but did not look at her for a while so
she could be free of my gaze. She started her bubbly chatter and I knew
we had moved along, together. She was starting to heal, so I was too.

I wrote a daily journal to Sarah during the chemo months. I wanted
her to have it whether I lived or died. Either way she might need it because I was sure that I would squash many things she might someday

want to know. I will give her the journal if and when she wants it. I have
just read it for the first time in order to help me write.

The journal records the details of my chemo regime and Sarah's re-
actions. I so wanted to make sure I gave Sarah the specifics she would
need of her experience of this time. I wanted her to know that at three
years old she was already a total person capable of loving and restoring
me daily. She stroked my bald head and would twirl the few wisps of
hair left; she insisted on washing my hair even though there was none;
she told me how she liked "pushed-in" breasts as much as regular ones.
She chose to think of them as pushed in rather than cut off. It wasn't
until she was almost ten that she asked me: "Mom, where did they throw
your breasts after they cut them off?" I remember realizing I had never
thought about this. I had never once wondered where my breasts were. I
cringed a bit when I answered her: "They were thrown away." It is significant that I never allowed myself this question and that she could.

The journal also depicts snatches of the rest of a three year old's life.
We discussed poverty and poor people, and Sarah wanted to know why
people have to be poor. We talked about the Bush/Dukakis presidential
race and Sarah decided to vote for Bush at the day-care election. She
loved embarrassing us with this information in front of her caregivers. I
have continued to write in the journal, though less regularly, and it gives
continuity to our memories.

Sarah is talking more about breast cancer but not very much. I tell
her each time I go for blood tracing, and she says it makes her worry but
that I must tell her anyway. I try to empower her and yet be honest. She
seems like an incredibly happy fifteen year old, in spite of all she has
been through. Or maybe her young experiences have made adolescence
easier to navigate. I really do not know. Clearly, there is no simple story
here. A few years ago when Sarah was terribly sick with a 105-degree
fever, she looked up at me and asked: "Do I have leukemia?" I assured
her that she was just sick, and also thought, why should she not wonder?

Sarah is now asking more about my sister Sarah. She often says how
much she wishes she had known her and how she misses her even
though she never knew her. The other day when Sarah asked me why

36 she was named Sarah I worried that maybe it is too difficult for Sarah to be named Sarah . . . but she protests that it is not. But I know that it is hard and that it is hard that I have had cancer and that Giah has died. Sarah finds that several of her friends do not want her to talk about this part of her life; they find it too sad.

Sarah, just now, is quite unsettled by her health course in school. She filled out a risk assessment form on breast cancer and her teacher told her she was at very high risk. Of course, this came as little surprise to Sarah, but she was terribly upset nonetheless. I have told Sarah that there are many kinds of risks, and that Sarah may be at less risk because of how she works at being healthy than someone who thinks she is not at risk and ignores health issues. Yet then I also say that her familial risk factor is real, and troublesome, and that I do not mean to deny her her fear, or my own.

I try to speak carefully what I think Sarah might be trying to think about but cannot quite voice. I cannot know what it feels like to be her age, to have known breast cancer her whole life, and to be receiving a new body as every girl at fifteen does. I so deeply believe that silence creates more fear that I continually try to open up the unknown however I can. I know that Sarah is working things through; her fear, her anger, and her love. She says that whenever cancer is discussed in her biology class her friend Alex tries to catch her eye to make her feel better.

Six months ago the phone rang and Sarah yelled to me that I needed to pick it up because it was Giah's doctor from Calgary calling. She stood there as I took the phone and heard the doctor tell me that the genetic testing of Giah had just been completed and she had the BRCA1 gene mutation. I felt so hollow to be told something about Giah that I could not tell her. I had assumed that she probably had the gene but somehow hearing that she did was a blow. I wondered whether her cancer had been written by this gene, or if this mutation just predisposed her to the cancer struggle, and whether it means I and Julia have the gene.

The strangest part was being defined through a gene pool as an ashkenazi jew when I am an atheist. This kind of racialized marking felt weirdly awkward; being defined beyond the self by this group identity in which I had no choosing.

Knowing Giah had the BRCA1 mutation makes everything seem more fixed than it is. Neither the safety nor the danger is a done deal. The gene is a predisposition but not for all women who carry it. I think you never know if it is the gene or the triggers to the gene that are the culprit.

Nevertheless, the gene is frightening. Julia and I discussed whether we should get tested. We had been putting off a decision. Now we knew Giah had it.

Julia decided to get tested. She wanted to be released from not knowing. She thinks that in some ways the testing is a win-win proposition. If she has the gene it shows her young nieces Sarah and Corenne that you can have the gene and be breast-cancer free at forty-five. If she does not have the gene, it means that you can be in a family like ours and not have inherited the gene. The tests are just back. Julia does not have the BRCA1 mutation.

I asked Sarah if she wants me to get tested. There is nothing left for me to do if I have the mutation, but the information will impact greatly on Sarah. If I have the gene, there is a fifty-fifty chance she has inherited it. This knowledge may just be too weighty at this moment in her life. But maybe she wants to be released from the anxiety of not knowing. Yet knowing may mean knowing that I have the gene.

Sarah said that she just "does not know whether she can know what to do." So I have decided, for now, not to be tested. When Sarah is in her early twenties we will revisit this issue unless she decides otherwise before then.

The other parts of Sarah move forward. She is more focused than I was at her age. She is very self-sufficient and self-determined. She readily identifies as a feminist and holds her own against the pressures of boy culture. She participated in the First National Girl's Conference held at the United Nations. She has read hundreds of books about children surviving the concentration camps in World War II and those who lived in hiding. So many children lost their parents in the war and yet they sur-

38    vived. So will she, if she has too. I think that she finds solace in their stories, that their collective identity soothes her. Right now she says she
wants to be a surgeon for Doctors Without Borders.

We began to deal more aggressively with a proactive diet for Sarah
when she started menstruating. All that we do is with measure because
otherwise it won't work for the long haul. We eat a low-fat diet, but she
loves cheese. I try to get her to eat whole grains with mixed success. She
now drinks a soy protein smoothy about four times a week, with a bit of
protest. She likes and is willing to eat tofu sandwiches for lunch. She is
pretty good about adding broccoli sprouts to salads and other foods. We
eat organic chicken. I try to have lots of fruits, especially in the summer,
but no strawberries, unless they are organic, because of high pesticide
use. She drinks skim milk that is not treated with rbST, and organic
cheese. She uses olive oil instead of margarines or butter.

Along with this I try to get her to do sports pretty regularly. Sarah ran
cross-country and plays racquetball and likes to canoe. She likes games
more than routine exercise, so her dad plays tennis with her. She likes to
win.

Last night, just before Sarah went to bed, she asked me if she could
have my chemo journal to read. I saw it on the floor next to her bed this
morning and took a deep breath.

# *My Other Bodies*

I AM UNEASY WITH THE STORY THAT EMERGES SO FAR. My family and I are more than our cancer narrative, and my body has other stories to tell. I need to write through my other bodies to find a fuller theorization. Theory is no abstract discussion for me. Instead it is a way of seeing and speaking how my female body is always in the process of becoming itself, through its fluid and plural history.

I do not see the female body as having a natural essence or some kind of true meaning. Rather, it is always embroiled with powerful cultural narratives and their psychic meanings. Bodies are intellectually and environmentally porous. Their borders are not simple or unchanging, and, therefore, neither are we.

I am writing to discover and reveal a bodily domain of power making. I am searching for a more complete expression of a female body because sites of power always begin with bodies. They are the starting

40 point of all meaning, and yet they never get to give meaning outside the power systems that already embrace them. My body offers me a "place-consciousness" from which to see experiences beyond myself.[1]

Female bodies are homogenized as though they are feminine and womanly at the start so to speak, which erases the very regulatory presumptions that demand the womanly depiction in the first place. So my body is completely personal and individual and unique *and* it is also universally seen as a woman's body. This tension is defined in and through a matrix that changes over time and space; across the life cycle, across a myriad of viewings with distinct historical and geographical and cultural locations.

Bodies tie females to one another because we share the same body no matter how differently. Yet each and every body is distinctly its own. It is this complete uniqueness and similarity that demand a theorization of female bodies as defining the "really real" of power and as a site for intimately local consciousness. "Really real" speaks to the materiality of the body rather than fantasy.

I am writing from my body, with my mind as a body part, from a sense not of self-importance but rather of discovery, believing that my body's story has further import. I am writing the personal—my bodies—to find its political meanings. This process of coming to consciousness about my body searches for the connective tissue defined by the power meanings that relate one body to another.

### Writing a Female Materiality

I want to write through to a materiality of the female body; or realities of female bodies. This materiality—which is also feminist—demands an understanding and theorization of female bodies in terms of their physicality and sexual desires *in* the structural constraints of a racialized class system. Most of my earlier writing has talked about the body from its outside. I now want to go inside and then come back out again. A female materiality must unveil and write a historical memory of the silenced meanings of this place-consciousness.

Writing from the body, my body, my different bodies, I have different stories to tell. They are all of a piece although they are also fragmen-

tary; as though each body experience has its own narration. In writing
my body/bodies there is no one complete story, but a multilayered history with no simple beginning, middle, or end. One's body makes several selves. As I open my body it reveals struggles with diabetes,
pregnancy, and a weakened postpartum self, menopause and aging,
muscle building and athleticism. My tales are in part made from my
flesh, and in part from my looking for them to tell of them.

The theorization of my body, as a start toward a female materiality,
seeks to create a memory in which I can see my body as an entire whole
in connection to the power-filled relations defining it, in order to move
through to the world made with these bodies. If I had a different body-
story, I might not have ever turned in this direction.

I am hesitant to name this theoretical project about female place-
consciousness and its materiality. I cannot find the right phrasing because no language quite fits my purpose. I am not simply speaking of an
economic-class-defined materialism like Marx, nor am I speaking of the
female body like french feminist Luce Irigaray.[2] But I do wish to particu-
larize the materiality of the female body as a uniquely compelling site
for resistance against human degradation and global obscenities.

There are uneasy translations and transitions from the personal body
to the political self; and from the political self to the personal body. This
subtly complex relationship sits at the heart of a fully defined sexual politics; there is a politics to sex and a sexual meaning to politics. The personal has political meaning and political meanings are personally lived.

There has never been any easy clarity about this connection. It is the
single most original theoretical insight of u.s. radical feminism: that the
female body is not one and the same with politicized femininity; that
sexual politics breaks open the public/private divide. However, this insight can be too solipsistic. To say that the personal *is* political reduces
each to the other. To say that the political *is* personal oversimplifies the
individualism of politics. But neither is it true that the personal is not
political; or the political is not personal.

To say that the personal is personal *and* political takes us to a variety
of meanings. Different bodily meanings have their own political effect.
But none of this complexity is embraced within popularized political
discourses. Only stolen fragments parade in the Clinton sex scandals,

42  the endless right-wing positioning on abortion, the querying of public officials about their private lives. All this distorts the complex political relations of bodies, their privacy, and their public meanings.

Feminist theory is a continual process of trying to make sense of the female body and what it has become without simply allowing biology to rule. Women are not simply their bodies, or simply victims of what they are kept from being, but are also what they are always trying to become. This is a more dynamic viewing of power; that oppression bespeaks potential power.

Simultaneously, popular culture and its entwining with mainstream politics make us all victims. Talk shows normalize betrayal, abuse, abandonment, sex trafficking, battering. The deradicalized feminist viewing of sexual oppression leaves us with a cultural language that speaks about sex without its politics.

So let me return to my body. My breast cancer body does not say enough about how other body demands have choreographed my life. Although breast cancer has often suffocated me and I have felt like there is almost no air to breathe, my body has had other selves. I am never simply my cancer because I have other bodies *and* I am something besides my body struggles. But meanings and discourses continually invade this process of knowing anything. I make myself think that I am never just my body, and yet I know my body can consume and destroy me.

It is hard to look backward and retell, try to really know my personal struggles with my body, just because I now want to know them. When I am seriously, actively inside the process of battling with my body, it tunnels me. I use all my energy to just fight back, and part of this fight numbs my brain. Then I am completely inside the process, and not looking at it.

### Body Tellings and My Writing

In my early twenties, active in the women's movement, and writing feminist theory, I did not consciously write my body. I had just finished the draft of the first chapter of my dissertation—which examined the

significance of Marxism for feminism—when I was severely injured in a    43
car accident.

I was on my way to dinner with friends to celebrate my writing of
this first chapter when a too young, sixteen-year-old new driver went
through a stop sign. I remember little of that night or the next few days.
My memory begins with the excruciating headaches from my fractured
skull and swollen brain. The stabbing pain from my broken ribs made it
impossible to rest. I was in the hospital for five weeks as I slowly began to
recover. I never fully healed, although the doctors thought I would with
time.

I lay in intensive care with white bandages covering my forehead
and face. My chin and neck had deep lacerations, and my forehead had
ballooned out into a grotesque form. I remember some of the first whis-
pers of friends beside my bed terrified at what they saw. My eyes were
blackened with internal bleeding. They worried that I would never be
the same.

My posterior pituitary gland was traumatized by the swelling of my
brain. Pitressin, which is the hormone normally secreted by this part of
the gland, stopped. Without it I became uncontrollably thirsty and
could not stop drinking water. Thirst consumed me; I could think of
nothing else but trying to stop the thirst. My nurses were frantic as I
gulped fifty gallons of water uncontrollably. I urinated clear water, washing my system of all the electrolytes it needed. I was lucky to have a
good doctor who realized pretty quickly what had happened. It was the
only case of diabetes insipidus he had ever seen.

Diabetes means thirst. The kind I have has nothing to do with sugar
diabetes (diabetes mellitus), which is caused by insufficient insulin secreted from the pancreas. The two illnesses just share symptoms.

It took months to regulate my medication. The first regime I was on
ruined my electrolyte count so I had to drink potassium chloride to try
and rebuild my electrolytes. The potassium wreaked havoc on my stomach. My breathing was often labored because the muscle around my
lungs was weakened by low electrolytes. I found all this horrifyingly difficult. I had lost my earlier carefree relationship to my body and I could
not find myself.

44    I was twenty-two years old at the time of the accident and it devastated me. I could not accept the stupidity of what had happened. I never felt lucky that I hadn't been killed. I actually never thought about death in this sense, but rather life itself now seemed utterly meaningless and irrational. What had happened to me was grotesque. My life was shattered forever. Purpose and control over what we do are simply a lie. I was sure that I or someone I loved would be killed in a car; or randomly taken for no good reason. I felt incapable of living with this new sense of loss. Living terrified me. I have often thought that I will never be destroyed by this truth again. Once it is known, it is known forever. But maybe not.

My Aunt Nettie was already sick when she traveled to Northampton to see me in the hospital. At that time we had not yet learned what was making her so ill. She made sure that she thought my medical care was good enough. She assured my mother and father that there was no need to have me moved to a New York City hospital.

I remember telling my mother that I no longer wanted to live, which is maybe slightly different from wanting to die. I can actually still feel the deadness of my feelings then. She just held me and I can also remember how the feel of her body challenged my sadness, awoke something inside me that I still wanted. Maybe right then I began to journey back; to start to try and fight the deadness, to begin to visit my new body demands, to begin again, with less fantasy. I began to try to know this new body; its labored breathing, its bruised bones and skull, its subtle warnings that I needed more medication.

I slowly reengaged with my life but cannot retrieve the process involved in getting me to do so. Looking back, I think my body's demands pushed me away from what I knew and I stopped thinking about death. I pushed death away not because I believed that it is not always there but rather because it is, and one lives knowing this but not thinking about it all the time. It is not helpful or useful to think about death once you put it inside the process of life. It feels boring and repetitive. I wanted to move through and beyond. Or maybe I just made my brain stop.

Again, I remember my beloved mother at this time. It was two months after the accident and she phoned. She was wondering how I was feeling, and I told her I was doing a little bit better. That I thought about dying much less, but that I didn't think that doing so resolves much. At first she was quiet and then said that she thought that I was healing, that not to think about death was all there was to do with it, that it was a healthy repression. I think she is right.

I have used a repressive stance other times as well. When I was in college one of my roommates got pregnant after always telling me she was not having intercourse. I helped her find a doctor. She was too frightened of the illegal abortions at that time to have one, so she left school, got married, and had the baby. I always have felt very sad about this. Many of my other college friends were often terrified they were pregnant. My solution to this was that I studied, kept boys and my feelings at a distance, and felt free. It worked through most of my college days. I never had a serious love affair until my senior year, but my fear of pregnancy was so strong that I was always extremely careful about using my diaphragm. I never got pregnant because I crafted a tight control. Looking back, I can romanticize a carefreeness that I wish I had had. But it is also this need for control over my body that kept me from taking the pill. The pill made me feel as if something other than myself was deciding about how I would use my body. I still wonder whether I too would have had breast cancer in my early twenties if I had taken it.

Dear Nettie had me come to the city and took me to a plastic surgeon she knew to see whether he thought my facial scars could be better camouflaged. I loved her for her concern and attention. My mother and father were so glad I was alive, they could have cared less about the facial scars. The surgeon, who at the time was mainly treating vietnam veterans, was incredibly honest and kind. He assured me that any surgery would leave me with some scarring, and that my stitching, if left alone, would fade with time. I looked at the maimed men in his office and thought how generous he had been to me. My face still has the contours of the initial stitching but it has just become my face.

My physical recovery was a slow and uninteresting process. I escaped to my dissertation. The writing process felt so purposeful; so much bigger than just my body. I did little else but study and write. I was singular in focus. Looking back to this time, I wonder if I was escaping

46 from the weakness of my body and whether I would have found this kind of concentration otherwise. It is impossible to know this, now.

I was writing feminist theory through my Marxist lens. Women's bodies were their labor. Later on, I would theorize the pregnant female body, but at this time and for a decade more I would imagine this body to be one and the same with its labor.

Women's labor, not their female bodies as such, was my fascination. Women's labor constructed them as one and the same with their reproductive (motherhood) and productive (wage-labor) and domestic (household and consumer) labor. For me at this time, the body, seen in terms of labor, is strong and productive, and not vulnerable. This did not mean that I was not viewing the oppressive conditions of factory labor, the electronics assembly line toxic hazards, migrant workers' horrid conditions, and so on. But I viewed this not from the body but from the place of work. It would take me many more years to look at the vulnerability of the body in my writing.

Although Marxist dialectics starts with real people as they inhabit their class, real people do not have "bodies" as such. For Marx, one is a member of a class and one's sex or gender or race is not theorized with autonomous or even semi-autonomous status. Although Marx mentions a first division of labor that derives from the sex act itself, all his theorization revolves around the second—economic class—division of labor.

Feminism starts from the self and moves outward but too often the self has not been dealt with in terms of one's body—the actual body of flesh and sexual desire.[3] Given that women have been so often reduced to their biological function, the body has long been considered a danger zone for feminists. Instead of engaging female desire and bodily needs, most political theory runs away. Equality with men (not male bodies) becomes the goal when one runs from the specifics of female bodies. We have moved from the personal and private realm of bodies to the public space of gender equality. When equality is said to mean the sameness of treatment, it is premised on the likeness between men and women, which leaves the particulars of the female body behind. Legal and economic equality stand in for the sexual body in sexual equality.

My Marxism demanded that I materialize—look directly at women's daily lives—and theorize power relations from this site. My Marxist familial origins had me placing and seeing the female body, not as a sexual and biological body, but as a construction of its economic class meaning, hence its labor. I was not going to theorize the body's vulnerability when this was exactly what my feminism rejected as biological determinism and my Marxism put outside my view. As a feminist, in my twenties, I very much thought that we are not our bodies, and as a Marxist I had little interest in this particular viewing of materialism.

As my body placed enormous constraints on me, and as I was learning to live within the limits of this new body, I was unable to embrace and look at this power of the body in my writing. I cannot be sure where I was in this process then. Looking back at myself in this way allows me to see the power of ideas and how they impact on the way we see, or do not see. This realization deeply affects my conscious reopening of my thinking today. My rethinking seeks to enrich and enlarge these earlier stances rather than reject them. And my body has demanded that I continually reopen myself to new possibilities.

As I wrote my way through to a dialogue between the Marxist understanding of labor specifically for women's waged and domestic activities and the radically feminist idea of women as a sexual class made up of females, I was determined to blend the systems of thought for each other's purposes. Sarah was already dying (1978) when *Capitalist Patriarchy and the Case For Socialist Feminism* was published.[4]

By then I followed my medical routine for the diabetes with little thought. There were days when the medication worked less well, but I was pretty adept at pushing it aside. I hated the checkups with the endocrinologist. His office was filled with terribly ill people, and I felt I was entering an entire world that healthy people never think about. Sitting in his office I was reminded of what I am always trying to forget. Bodies are incredibly limiting.

Sarah was fighting for her life, but I loved her too much to consciously say that that was what she and we were doing. I just kept dealing with each day—not looking forward most of the time. I knew she was going to die but I did not, and I would not let myself think about it, so I did not let myself know.

48 Sometimes, on a good day, I would write to create another reality, and it was a comfort. When my own body was still coming back to its former strength and while Sarah was fighting a virulent metastasis to her lung and brain, I wrote about the creative potential of women's labor. We were not just our bodies. The structural meaning of patriarchal privilege was found not in women's individual bodies as simply female, but in their labor both inside and outside the paying economy. I was demanding a viewing of female bodies in their structural/politically economic meanings, not simply as female flesh or potential childbearers. I still deeply believe this labor is crucial, but it is only one expression of our bodies' political materiality.

I wrote *The Radical Future of Liberal Feminism* (1981) in the period shortly after Sarah's death.[5] My writing was my form of meditation. I began to break through my earlier blinders and wrote of women as a sexual class, displacing the singularity of the notion of class as an economic category. I used the Marxist focus on labor to uncover the revolutionary potential of feminism even in its bourgeois form. As more and more women entered the labor force, women's doubled class realities—economic *and* sexual—would mobilize a consciousness of the double day of work for women.

I was mourning Sarah and celebrating the revolutionary potential of women as I wrote. Even mainstream feminism had enormous potential, in my mind, to unsettle politics as usual. The strength of the women's movement at this time seemed hopeful. And I was shattered and bereft at the loss of my beloved older sister.

## Body Memory and Body Knowing

I am writing in the hopes of retrieving more meanings of my body in order to have a body memory which can let me know how we come to be who we are. It has taken me time to look back and try to see more clearly from this place.

So I am searching for memory when memory itself is a construction. I know I do not remember everything, so I must be remembering what I

allow myself, what I wish to remember. Maybe there is no such thing as    49
real memory of real pain, and I simply think I remember what I did not
know. I know part of living is making oneself forget. Sometimes forgetting is called forgiveness. For me, I know it is that I have simply forced
myself to forget. I am not thinking about seeing my sadness when I am
in too much pain. So maybe if I can write of my sorrow and loss, this
means that I have become someone else in this process, someone who is
more healed and distant. Maybe I have just forgotten enough to let myself try and remember.

For many years I never wondered about the physicality of my writing
process. Today, I keep having to get up and drink water . . . and pee . . .
while writing. Either thinking about the diabetes makes me conscious of
what I do unconsciously every day—drink and pee more than most people—or I am having one of my bad medication days; or my brain is unsettling my body.

Even though I live consciously with my body almost every day, I also
push away from it daily. So my political writing is more about my body
than I have been able to recognize, but it is not just a dialogue with my
body. Routes are circuitous and simultaneously sedimentary. So I look
through my body not to find it standing alone as some kind of explanation or cause but rather to find how my body becomes dispersed in and
through a variety of locations. Biology is not destiny, and it sometimes is
everything.

When I wrote *The Female Body and the Law* (1985–88) in a postpartum body, I never thought I was writing from my body at the time.[6] I
wrote of the female body and its dismissal and negation through law
while my own body was still healing from pregnancy and childbirth. I
wrote of the pregnant body as a legal dilemma given the law's silenced
masculinist standard. I argued that the female body must be pluralized
to the reality of bodies; and this radically nonstandardized starting point
must rewrite legal discourse itself.

Birthing Sarah at the age of thirty-seven with my diabetes pushed my
body almost beyond what it could do. It took several years to rebuild my
physical stamina. But none of this made its way into my writing. I wrote

50  politically, not personally, about pregnancy. The female body was not
one and the same with my body or Sarah's or Giah's or Julia's. It was a
decade after Sarah had died and Giah had fought off two breast cancers.

I had decided in my mid-twenties that I would probably not have
children. I had no compelling desire to do so. I liked the life I was living
and did not want to change it. Because of the car accident, my doctors
were not sure I could get pregnant anyway. They knew that my posterior
pituitary did not function, and were not fully sure about the anterior
part, which is necessary for ovulation. It remained unclear whether I
was regularly ovulating. Maybe my injured body played more of a role
here than I understood at the time. I cannot know this now.

My mother played an important role in my thinking in this realm
too. In conversations I had with her while I was in graduate school—before the car accident—I asked her how I would ever know whether I
should have a child or not. I would always say how much I loved what I
was doing, and wondered if I would be really happy having a baby and
raising a child. She, a woman who knows how to deeply love her children, would always say that if I was hoping not to change my life in
major ways, I should leave it as it was. She had no qualifiers. Her complete confidence gave me new resolution to just be myself. When I
think back to this time I am amazed at how incredible she was. She had
no need for me to be anything other than what I wanted. I did not return
to this issue of parenting for a very long time. Sarah's death left me
frightened of life's commitments. After she died I did not want to have to
love deeply again.

But life is so much more complicated than I could ever allow myself
to imagine in advance. After separating from the man I had lived with
for many of the years I have just written about—I met Richard. At first I
thought it was impossible for anyone who had not met me before the car
accident and Sarah's death to ever really know me. I wanted Richard to
know me as I was before Sarah and my father's death, before I was who I
have become. This being impossible, I found myself searching for ways
to discover and refind the parts of life that would open me again. My
new passionate energy with Richard had us thinking about getting preg-

nant. Richard was completely devoted to trying to have a baby and to  51
keeping me safe through it.

My doctors thought that if I could get pregnant it might still take a
very long time to do so. They were wrong. I got pregnant almost too
soon. I still remember that great moment when the home pregnancy
test turned red. I felt I was beginning an unknowable journey. I was not
at all fearful of the process, just totally determined to make my body
work.

I had already switched from the synthetic diabetes medication I was
taking to the natural form of pitressin by injection. My endocrinologist
at first thought the pitressin injections would be too difficult for me to
manage and that the synthetic medication I was taking would probably
not affect the fetus. But Doctor Streeton could not really know this
given the rarity of my condition, so he was unable to ease my concern.
In the end he agreed to teach me how to inject the natural form of
pitressin.

I would need an injection about every twelve hours. It is oil based
and must be given intramuscularly. The needle has to be long enough
to go deep into the muscle, and it must be thick enough for oil to pass
through it. The oil has to be heated just before shooting it. Streeton
showed me first how to prepare the injection and then to insert the needle into an orange for practice . . . and then I sat staring at my thigh . . .
unable to enter it. I sat, trying to tell myself to do it, and just sat. I sat and
stared for what seemed like forever. And then, by forcing myself not to
think, I made my hand push through my skin and slowly probe down
into my muscle. This process never got easy. My thighs still are etched
by the scarring from the oil deposits.

Three-quarters of the way through the pregnancy my legs could not
absorb the injections anymore. Richard started injecting me in the hip.
My body also became more erratic in is use of the pitressin. I often
could not stretch the dose for more than six hours. I would then rush
out of my office to Richard's as I could feel my body's thirst increasing,
warm the pitressin, get the shot, breathe deeply, and return to work.

With all this difficulty, I was still running five miles a day. I actually

52  ran the day I delivered. Running is my form of controlling my out-of-control body. It is how I rebuilt myself after the accident. There are several bodyselves here; and also only one.

Writing about this period is very strange because the pregnancy looked at from the outside bears little resemblance to the physical experience of being pregnant. Looking back, I wonder how I did it; I could never do it now. Back then, the process itself enveloped me. My body demanded that I not think about my body. I narrowed my brain waves and used them to make my body work. Richard and my beloved friends had a harder time with their worry. They were watching and looking and thinking. I was just living it.

Now, when I think I could not do it again, it means that because I do not have to, I cannot think that I could. Necessity is amazing. It is what brought me through the childbirth itself.

My body was stretched to its limits in birthing. Labor went on for too many hours. Early on the pain was violently located in my back. After fifteen hours I had no sense of separate body parts. I had trouble holding onto a sense of conscious awareness. After delivery I was bleeding heavily and my exhaustion reached deep into each piece of my flesh. There was no ecstasy, but instead release from the pain, and then fear of the damage just done to my body.

I remember thinking, I have done it, and now I must rest. My body did not feel like the one I had known in pregnancy; this body was not mine. I did not know this body and I was frightened. Richard was petrified for me and crying but held his newborn daughter in his arms. He named her Sarah the minute he saw her finally emerge. When we spoke of names early on I did not know if my daughter could have my sister's name. I deeply loved him for choosing her name that moment. He pushed her around in her nursery cart and fed her her first bottle.

Sarah had ripped through the episiotomy. It took Joyce almost an hour to sew me up. I faded in and out of consciousness, not feeling part of the world. I thought, I will try to breast-feed tomorrow. I will do nothing more today. I can do nothing more. All I want to do is sleep; to forget my wrecked body. Maybe when I wake I will be strong again. Sarah is here and I am done.

My body did not allow me to feel triumphant. It was too weak. As I    53
tried to sleep I kept feeling too emptied. As I bled I wondered if I could
make yet one more body recovery. I had no idea that night or the next
several months how long the rebuilding would take. Maybe I just would
not let myself know. The aftermath of pregnancy—the beat-up vaginal
walls, the sagging uterus, the extra stomach flesh, the post-breast-fed
breasts, the thicker waist, my low electrolyte count—meshes with the
entire process of my aging body.

Richard and I were parenting Sarah and working at life. She was not
a sleeper so neither were we. We fantasize sleep each day. I was running
again though my uterus was lower. It is with this body that I wrote *The
Female Body and the Law*, but I was nowhere near claiming my body as
part of my thought process.

Time passed. I was diagnosed with breast cancer and did several surgeries and chemo. I continued, when I could, to radically pluralize the
specificity of the female body in my writing. I racialized the construct of
female bodies in *The Color of Gender* (1994).[7] The revolutions of 1989
and the Reagan-Bush decade demanded my engagement with democratic theory. Debates within the women's movement about its whiteness, the political assault against affirmative action law for people of
color and white women, the lack of a public health approach to AIDS,
turned me to exploring the racial meanings of the female body.

I then argued that not only does the female body need to be specified for retheorizing democratic imaginings but these bodies must name
racial privilege along with pregnancy. I imagined beyond my whiteness
to black women who may be pregnant and argued that they should be
the starting point for democratic theory. Meet their needs and everyone's needs will be met as a result. Their specificity will become the
new route for demanding a truly democratic universality. I wrote from
outside my own body, again, while my body had brought me here.

The wars in bosnia and rwanda were the focus of my next work. I
traveled to bosnia to meet with women who were against the war. I did-
n't want to but I found myself writing *HATREDS* (1996). I kept wondering why bodies and especially women's bodies are the sites for horrific
hatred. I examined the way that nationalism is written with the war-rape

54 of women's bodies. I wrote of race as a particular construction of physicality—through color, hair, noses, vaginas—and patriarchy as a system of masculinist power became a completely racialized system of power for me.

My own body had been cut and was still healing from chemo. I still never thought if my own body impacted on the writing I was doing. My body was molded by illness and disease while I was writing about and looking at bodies etched by hatred. I think, however, that my body has opened me to these sadnesses elsewhere. When I traveled to bosnia and met with women who were raped in the name of ethnic cleansing, I knew, in my own way, that they wanted to leave their bodies behind and could not. I do not mean to parallel my experience with theirs, but to use it as a site of connection.

My mind continued to traverse the changing political relations of global capital. The u.s. is said to be the most economically unequal country in the world with its highs and lows, and I began to return to my more Marxist days. But my return was different because of my body that had made its own journeys. So I rethought the way that global capitalism highlights and exacerbates the class differences among women, in the u.s. and abroad, in terms of labor *and* I began to think about their bodies' health. I wrote *Global Obscenities* (1998).[8] I was angered at the way women, and especially girls, are targeted as the cheapest form of labor in electronic and garment factories across the globe and how their breast tissue is compromised. I scoffed at the prosthetic promises of cyberspace, as though our bodies can matter less in a world that is so economically, and racially, and sexually exploitative.

Giah was diagnosed with ovarian cancer as I was working on *Global Obscenities*. I had my ovaries removed and did yet one more surgery. I hated the scar from this operation more than the mastectomy scars. I felt that I was losing my body parts and that not enough of me would be left. I was critiquing cybercapitalism's exploitation of women while living through Giah's death as a constant reminder that without our bodies we die.

I also found myself seeing and writing more about girls and their health as my own daughter has became a teenager. I find myself spending

more and more time with her as she tries to negotiate her world. She  55
seems to feel so displaced by her changing body and by schools that feel
too prison-like to her. I know she will get through this but it is not easy.

### Retheorizing Bodies as Traveling

Let me try and start all of this a bit differently. I am always wondering what it means to "really" think and therefore "really" live responsibly
and creatively. My ideas continually evolve and change and go backward and then forward again. My thinking and writing and teaching and
public/political life are all of one process. There are basic themes I have
devoted my life to but they have taken different paths at different personal and political and historical moments. My body writes different stories and a story is written from my different bodies.

I moved to Ithaca to teach at Ithaca College over a quarter of century ago. I was twenty-four years old my first year of teaching. At this
time the u.s. women's movement was at its most radical stage, and I
taught feminist theory. Some of the members of the all-male department that I joined were hesitant to hire me. They told me later on that
they had worried I would be too difficult to get along with.

When I look back at this period I can see that I was still recuperating
from my car accident, but I did not know that then. You cannot know
that your body will get stronger and heal more. I just lived in the body I
had.

I taught differently, then than now, because times were different. We
were still in the aftermath of the civil rights and black power movement,
the feminist movement was both mainstream and insurgent, the global
economy was just beginning to consolidate itself. It was before the re-
structuring of labor—in the academy and outside—and in the aftermath
of downsizing. My ideas and writing and teaching continued to engage
and disengage with the demands of these shifting times.

I ask my students and myself to remain uncomfortable with their
knowledge, seeking new modes of rethinking, reseeing, and acting
courageously. I try to displace myself . . . remove my sense of home, and
homelands. My body has pushed me in this direction. The insecurities

56  of my physical body narrow and broaden me. I fight this narrowness each day, and sometimes am defeated, other times not. I am most able to push outside myself when my body gives me the reprieve to do so. Just now, my sense of openness toward looking *at* my body is possible because I am not consumed by a new struggle with it. I grab this fanta-sized security to look inward and to explore elsewhere.

I often think that the lack of guaranteed health care and health in-surance is the most incredible form of political control and regulation that exists. This lack is a continual reminder to each of us of our own vulnerabilities. The needs of the body can smash through anything and everything.

I travel to displace and unsettle myself from the outside. I leave home, so to speak, to experience variety. My struggle to control and know my body, which keeps changing on me, curtails the ability to de-sire the unknown. Yet I try to overcome this need by unsettling myself through the unfamiliar. I travel beyond the globalized familiarity to open myself up again and again. My recent travel, to bosnia and cuba and ghana remind me of the confines of my geographical and bodily culture. Sometimes one need not go far. When my family and I entered the Ghana Airways terminal at Kennedy Airport there was not a white person to be seen. We had already become differently conscious of our-selves and had not yet used our passports.

### *"Really Real" Bodies*

Knowing, seeing, and naming have become more difficult as I in-habit a world that is more image than real; where truth has little politi-cal status but depends, as then-president Clinton said, on what the meaning of "is" is. Or, as the talented Mr. Ripley (in the 1999 film of the same name) reveals: "I always thought it would be better to be a fake somebody than a real nobody." I want to find the "really real" while real fakes dominate our mental landscapes.

So my process of thought is still dedicated to the theorization—the connected seeing and viewing—of the structural relations of racialized class patriarchal power, but I take my body more knowingly with me.

For me, theory demands connecting the dots: seeing connection, relationship, woven sections, processes without clear borders; from body to nation to globe. Theory stands counter to and in subversion of the individualist discourse of neoliberalism that dominates today. Supposedly individuals can change their lives for the better if they wish. Each of us is responsible for who and what we become—our health and our well-being are our own responsibility.

In this vision there is no structural racism, or sexism, or class-based power: individuals own their power. And although there is a bit of truth here, it is becoming less and less true as economic disparity grows. Meanwhile millions more of us are medically uninsured and less healthy than in years past.

Part of the trouble in really seeing and understanding is that the discourses that surround us and enter us demand that we think individually, selfishly, singularly, and in the moment—while also denying the urgency of the body. There is little history as memory; there is little sense of the whole, but rather simply the parts. I want to build walkways that let us see/act subversively, with our bodies, as part of this process of really seeing and acting on this place-consciousness.

My writing and teaching are now dedicated to unraveling and finding the constantly changing economic structures of racialized patriarchal body parts. To theorize patriarchy is to see how sex is transformed into gender and gender back into sex, so that it is both impossible to see the difference between being born female and becoming a woman and also completely necessary to know that this distinction exists. But becoming a woman—adopting one's gender—is simultaneously defined in and through one's economic class beginnings, and one's class is deeply tied to one's race. This is so while one's color is treated as though it were the same as race, and it is not. But let us take this all into the breast and take the breast into these meanings. The breast has visibility in a way the uterus does not. The breast speaks sexual desire, maternal feeding and mammies, and the objectification of females, reducing them to their bodies.

These processes shift and change as the u.s. moves from industrial capitalism to a service economy tied to a global network. These structural

58 changes make it harder to see the intersections betweeen race and sex and class as they define the body, while bodies impact on these meanings. *And* the systems are not separate and apart. But I think that the bodies of women connect them to each other while all else may seek to sever this connection. If this is so, women's breasts can help us write and create a newly democratized politics.

The uniqueness of feminisms—that they must start with the self, the personal, the body, and work outward, beyond the self to the shared meaning of this starting point—makes clear that our bodies function as *signs* before we have been allowed to give them our own personal and individual meaning. One becomes a feminist as one recognizes the shared meaning of being female in the world; however one constructs the `idea' of being a female in one's individual body it stands counter to a prescribed enforced meaning of womanhood. If one sees only oneself, in singular fashion, there is no knowing that we, as female bodies, share a similar location of being women, defined in and through patriarchal regimes and practices that ascribe us meanings other than what we are and think ourselves to be. Seeing similarity means that we can see through the varieties of ascribed and chosen meanings to this shared— but not identical—space.

The similarities are not unified or equivalent to sameness. Women are both similar and different; similarly different and differently similar. So are our bodies and our breasts. Race and economic class differentiation make this more true.

My meaning of racialized patriarchy focuses the system of male privilege on its negotiations by and through racialized meanings. Gender is already racialized—masculinity is color-coded, while race is engendered—women of color are colored while whiteness is neutralized. So is breast tissue.

The process is not one of unity or simply differentiation. Patriarchy is the differentiating of women from men while privileging men *and* the transformation of females to women and males to men in this process. Yet gender is differentiated in racism, and racism is differentiated by race *and* gender. Racialized patriarchy roots male privilege in racism

*and* racism is differentiated by race *and* gender. I readily admit that the 59
term *"and"* is not quite right because bodies reconnect and weave
through this.

The state is no longer envisioned as simply harmonizing nation-
based interclass conflict but rather as assisting the mobility of global
capital and its racial borders. These processes take place in and through
real bodies. The imaginary globe sometimes replaces and sometimes
just simply coexists with the imagined economic nation. The overlap
between globe and economic nation allows for a continual privatization
of the political nation. Citizens are then simply a new kind of consumer. And the nation-state becomes a significant player in the process
of globalizing capital while giving new license to its racial-sexual formation. We are left to cope with our bodies ourselves.

As such, statist patriarchy is re-formed as a transnational gendered
division of labor of the information age. Women's exploitation is rewired
at computer terminals throughout countries of the south and north.
Global patriarchy is oftentimes less directly sustained through the privatized nation-state than through the numbing inequalities of the market
and the challenges this poses for our bodies. However, the privatized nation-state *is* a state policy, though a negative one, which also helps to
sustain capitalist racialized patriarchy.

Patriarchal privilege relocates itself in new formulations of the public and private, and nation and family nexus. It means that masculinist
privilege operates through a series of signs that are actually disconnected
from their earlier historical forms and points of origin. The new forms of
racialized patriarchal privilege written into transnational globalism are
tied both to traditional signs of femaleness and to newer media-ted fantasies of privatized governments.

## Locating Bodies with Their Power

The cyberreal of racialized gender presents the labor of women and
girls in the prosthetic language of Microsoft and transnational media
corporations. I seek to refind the bodies *and* their labor to dismantle the

60 mystifying fantasy of the supposed disembodied global culture. Cyber-language says there is no center, no power, no race or gender, no one owning in the so-called old way. The only thing that is said to matter is knowledge and one's embrace of one's new, classless, raceless, gender-less freedom. The cyberscreen is the free market where the limitations of the body supposedly no longer matter.

In actual fact, cyberspace is a construction of digital apartheid, a newly actualized form of racial exclusion. Most countries in Africa fall off the global map if electricity and phone lines are necessary. Given that only one in five people across the globe has a phone line, the internet becomes an exclusive suburban community. Yet this is not perfectly true.

Tragically, just as telecommunications *could* hook up the world, no commitment exists to create the equality of access that could make this happen. Instead, new technologies rewrite and expand new inequalities on top of those that already exist. As we speak of information highways, we need to remember that one out of three women worldwide is illiterate and spends a significant portion of her day performing essentials like collecting firewood and drawing water. Cyberspace will simply remain a new kind of country club if unchallenged.

The illusion of reality cannot be allowed to substitute for reality. Power and oppression are not simply signs with no origin. Cyberlanguage, then, expresses a politics of body and mind, labor and technology. It is imperative, then, to see that global capital and its cyberdiscourse obfuscate the real: the racialized patriarchal division of labor that disproportionately locates women and girls in low-wage assembly and information jobs and in sexual ghettoes elsewhere in the global market while making their bodies invisible.

Women are half of humanity and remain the poorest of the poor. We do approximately two-thirds of the world's work and earn about one-tenth of the world's income. We own less than one-hundredth of its property. We make up a majority of the world's refugees. We attempt to make life possible while living in degraded environments. We are the best hope to stand against the obscene agenda of transnational capitalist/racialized patriarchy because it is destroying our bodies: in nationalist

wars, in the workplace, in religious fundamentalist assaults, in crass corporatist commercialism, and in contaminated breast milk and breast
tissue.

## A Breast-Felt Politics

Cyberdiscourse gives us prosthetics rather than bodies. But bodies
are too *real*. Anyone who is hungry knows the *realness* of the body. Anyone who has fought disease knows this. We are stuck with our bodies.
Feminism, as a politics that is committed to theorizing the body as a site
of resistance, must return from the cyberglobe to this problematic place.

I do not mean to say that women are only their bodies, or even
mainly their bodies, or that our bodies give us a special essential meaning that men cannot have. Rather, I mean simply to say that female bodies—especially breast tissue—absorb their environs in unique ways that
need to be theorized and politicized. Women carry the polluted globe
around in our bodies, especially in our breast tissue and breast milk.

Feminism's contribution here is that once gender and race (and sex
and color) are denaturalized as not simply genetic/biological constructions, then breasts themselves, as part of female bodies, are viewed as
open environments absorbing contaminated air and cultural predisposi-
tions. Such a viewing is a quite different scenario from that of a biogenetically determined breast cancer . . . or the bodiless fantasy of
cybercapitalism.

I am neither a biological determinist nor an environmental one. I
respect and fear each. But now I have brought you to my present writing, which directly addresses the body through the breast with cancer. I
have exposed my body—from the inside out and the outside in—as a
place for progressive resistance.

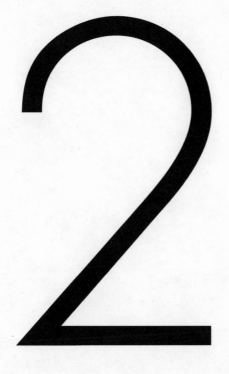

Politicizing the Personal

# Theorizing a Breast Cancer Gene

I NEVER IMAGINED I WOULD THEORIZE ABOUT
breast cancer.

Although I begin from the local site of my body, there is no one
starting place, no one node, so to speak, for this project.

I begin with a series of nodal points that overlap and layer into themselves. I use "node" to mean a thick intersection of multiple tangents
creating a messy knot. Knots can be unwound but most often not neatly.
These nodal knots initiate and also continuously reopen my thought
process.

Because cultural and political thought is complexly layered into the
practices of science, scientists are not separate from—do not live apart
from—the racialized and gendered and classed ways of seeing. I wish for
a critically scientific stance that always looks for multivalent complex
activity. The interplay between the body's health and its political, and

66     cultural, and scientific surroundings demands an honest skepticism and
       scrutiny. Do not misunderstand me here. I believe in scientific method
       and discovery, but not in the singularized causal sort that silences more
       than it reveals.

       Too many narratives of breast cancer, which parade scientifically,
       are not simply about breast tissue per se. There are powerful financial
       and political thought systems that construct breast cancer research and
       treatment. Because of this, breast cancer is always, at least in part, politi-
       cally articulated. I wish to displace the ruling narratives and the natural-
       ized silences they imbibe with a more complex dialogic of multiple and
       overlapping environments that dislodge the usual parameters of cause
       and effect.

       The very language I use to query and investigate the master narra-
       tives of breast cancer is imbricated in the systems of thought I wish to
       challenge. So I have no new truth to share, but rather wish to demythol-
       ogize the scientific stance of truth. Much less is scientifically known
       about female biology than is presented to women. Anyone who has
       been pregnant knows how inexact the knowledge base is here: due
       dates, weight gain, fetal nutrition, postpartum depression. Estrogen re-
       placement is hard to figure out because there is so little established
       knowledge of uniquely female body activities.

       This does not mean that I do not recognize the reality of breast can-
       cer cells or their unrelenting determinative status once they are in
       process. As one fights for one's life against breast cancer, biology can feel
       like destiny. In such moments all one wants to know is cause, and cure.
       I still dream about a cure for breast cancer before my daughter turns
       twenty. It is what I wish for every time birthday candles are blown out.
       In my less dreamy private moments I know that something will have to
       change radically before this happens. So I think about the nodal knots
       and how to untie and weave them together.

       *Node* 1. Breast cancer is both an individual and a socially and politi-
       cally constructed experience. Breast cancer is intimate and public; per-
       sonal and political; genetic and environmental; economic and
       racialized; local and global.

       *Node* 2. Breast tissue begins to form by the fourth week of fetal life.[1]

Mythologies of the breast are already in place at the time of birth.
Breasts are always part fantasy while they are also flesh. The phantas-
matic perfect breast shimmers across our culture for all women to see.

Node 3. Because the racialized viewing of womanhood privileges
whiteness and white women as the symbol of beauty, the breast as the
object of beauty becomes white. To the extent that the breast is imaged
as white, breast cancer also becomes imaged as white. Most drug trials
are of white middle-class women. Most breast cancer studies are of this
same population.

Node 4. Breast cancer has many faces that are not readily in view.
Women with breast cancer in rwanda, kosovo, turkey, and south africa,
and the millions of women living as refugees across the globe, struggle
with the violence of war and their lack of access to any health care.
Women in iraq and cuba suffer the consequences of u.s. embargoes and
economic sanctions, making most detection and treatment of breast disease impossible.

Node 5. My chest is now a strong wall of muscle with two thin lines
stitched closed where my breasts used to rest. When I look at my chest I
seldom think about my breasts; and I do not not think about them.
Maybe I just think I do not think.

My breasts were amputated but I do not feel mutilated. I fought
against thinking my body had been disfigured, but I do not remember
having to work hard at this. I built a new chest and rejected implants.
My path was to build my own muscle and create sexual/sensual pleasure
on this new terrain.

My family, my friends, and my feminism filled the new absences on
my chest. I was different after the surgeries, but also not so different. I
became who I became.

I am bothered by JoAnne Motichka, the artist whose chest graced
the front page of the *New York Times Magazine* shortly after her mastectomy, who has won a two-million-dollar suit against her surgeon for the
unnecessary "mutilation" of her body. To me, mutilation means that you
can no longer recognize the person that once was there. I would have
sued for malpractice if I thought the surgery was unnecessary, not mutilation. I obviously see a breastless chest differently than she does. Many

68    women who have chosen preventive breast surgery without reconstruction appear to feel similarly to me.[2]

   *Node 6*. Dominant and popularized discourses of breast cancer, often parading as scientific, disinform as much as inform, create false closure when openness is needed, narrow rather than broaden options for understanding the multicomplexity of the breast. Neither disease nor medical knowledge is simply biological in its construction, because they overlap with the wider values and conditions of society. Breast disease is a mix of combinations that are already culturally and politically in place.[3] All this needs unpacking in order to scrutinize the terrorizing fear created by the dominant narratives.

   *Node 7*. Breast cancer reflects and also constructs the medicalized gender visors of the historical moment. These social constructions shift and change within the patriarchal visionings of the female body. Gender, as it defines visions of womanhood, transcends and becomes a part of the female body. Nancy Krieger and Elizabeth Fee say that gender, as a social reality, can even transform our biology.[4] Breasts make the woman, and breast cancer is thought through and within this field. Racism is encoded here, once again, in and through a racialized construction of gender.

   *Node 8*. Most breast cancer narratives conceive of the female body as driven by estrogen. Cancer cells, fed by estrogen, are viewed as self-determining rather than as a complex multifarious process of long-term mutations that interact with the body and its environments. The environment enters our body and does not remain outside. Instead, our body is the environment for our cells; molecules provide the environment for atoms; atoms for protons. But more on this later.

   *Node 9*. Most women deeply fear breast and ovarian cancer. Yet one woman dies every minute across the globe from causes related to pregnancy and childbirth. For every one of these deaths, at least thirteen others suffer a less serious threat to their health.[5] More women die from heart disease than breast cancer, yet it is breast cancer that women seem to fear most.

   *Node 10*. Breast cancer exists within and alongside the discourses of the established medical-postindustrial complex. This complex defines

the contours of the cancer establishment as well as reflects the dem; ıds
of a transnational medicalized corporate structure. All this complicates
the possibilities of imagining and creating a science free to explore a
holistic, interactive, and preventive modeling of the disease.

My thinking is knotted through these multiple nodes, which creates
a rhizomed layering of my thought. Rhizomes are thick meandering
horizontal stems that store food and assist reproduction of new life.
Their meanderings, and storage, and horizontal webbing allow for my
continual opening and reopening of the breast against its silences. I am
looking to create new healthy growth for seeing differently and building
a place-consciousness of resistance.

## Knotting the Breast to Its Construction

One is not born with breast cancer. One develops it. It grows over
time. It has a history, inside, through, and outside our bodies.

The prevalence of the disease appears to be increasing. A woman
has about a 10 percent cumulative probability of developing breast cancer in her lifetime if she lives to eighty-five, and this chance increases
with age.[6] Since 1960 more than 950,000 women have died from breast
cancer.[7]

One is also not born with developed breasts, but rather with breast
tissue and ducts. Next breast buds develop. Then breasts grow and
change further. Breast tissue appears to be more vulnerable to damage
from carcinogens, pesticides, radiation, biopsy needles, and so on.
There is some thought that breasts may be more susceptible to carcinogens than other parts of the body.

Breast cancer is played out on and through a terrain that is politicized by an extremely sexualized symbolic of womanhood. In masculinist visions women are often reduced to their bodies via their breasts and
collapsed into their sexual/sensual selves. Female breasts identify the
woman's body. They also may provide milk and sustain life, and they
may not. They are deeply woven into one's bodily identity, and yet I can
live without them if I must. Breasts, as central to the symbolic phantasm
of womanhood, become both real and fantasy. Breasts are enormously

70    significant because they are made so *and* because of their physicality
and sensuality, which are in part always in combination with the fan-
tasy-real.

Dominant narratives of breast cancer—scientific and lay—construct
*and* reflect masculinist culture, which objectifies and fetishizes the
breast. These power-filled fantasies are often indistinguishable from the
cultural aspects of science itself. The fantasized perfect breast—which
few women have without surgical augmentation—underlies an often
cosmetic approach to the disease. Preventive mastectomies are not covered by most health insurance policies, while reconstructive surgery
after mastectomy usually is.

Breasts are sexual organs; yet they are also fetishized as commodity
parts. So they are an integral wonderful part of the female body and also
commodified in exploitative and dehumanizing ways. Mastectomy
treats the breast as disposable; lumpectomy cherishes it. Neither is de-
void of cultural implication. Mastectomy, amputation of the breast, was
the surgery used through the 1970s with breast reconstruction through
implants, instituted more recently, as the common postmastectomy procedure. Breast conservation, lumpectomy, is now the procedure most
widely used by doctors. There is statistical data to prove that it is similarly effective to mastectomy.

Either medical procedure must be chosen recognizing the complicated needs each person has. Although lumpectomy is usually a sufficient procedure, sometimes it may not be. Although mastectomy is most
often not necessary, sometimes it may be. Breast conservation, though
fought for by breast cancer health activists and heralded by Dr. Susan
Love, does not operate on neutral ground, because there is no neutral
ground. Each individual woman needs to make her own choice, when
her own particular history is never one and the same with statistical
probability. One's thinking about one's body is crucial in deciding on
one's health. Neither procedure frees the woman from the phantasmat-
ics of breast culture.

My female oncologist, who recommended mastectomy for me,
could not discuss mastectomy without speaking about breast reconstruction. The two were intimately connected for her and the cosmetic

outcome enormously important. Although she thought recurrence was
a likely possibility, given my family history, she was less driven by this
concern. We differed greatly on this.

The strands building the nodal knots intertwine repeatedly. Breast
cancer is bodily, individual, and intimate. And it also operates within a
patriarchal, capitalist, racist, and consumerist society that plays a part in
defining the disease in the first place. Genes and estrogen tell too little
of this story. Studies and drug trials must focus on more varied popula-
tions of women in order to see the unique and shared qualities of estrogen. After all, "all humans share approximately 95 percent of their
genetic makeup."[8]

Because breast cancer plays out in such devastating ways for individual women, the dominant focus is on individual detection and treatment, personal coping, and so on. At a local meeting hosted by the
Ithaca Breast Cancer Alliance, set to discuss diet and the lower levels of
breast cancer in rural china, every question asked of the epidemiologist
who was presenting dealt with what individual women can do to change
their diet here, in the u.s. This response is understandable but also problematic, because breast cancer is lived societally *and* individually. One
cannot simply translate the multienvironmental issues of breast cancer
into an individual choice of diet. The connection between the personal
and the environmental aspects of breast cancer is not one of equiva-
lence. No one factor can address the complexity.

Women need to recognize that there probably is no individual solution to this problem for now, and that an individualist and singular kind
of seeing will not create the spectacularly revelatory science needed. In
the interim, I too grow broccoli sprouts and eat natural grains and tofu.
The personal will always matter even if it does not change things
enough. Meanwhile we must continue to travel back and forth from the
personal into the political.

## Manmade CancerCapitalism

The racialized sexual politics of breast cancer and woman's breasts
complicate health care in a political and economic system that has little

72   commitment to protecting and insuring the health of the public. The prevalent medical discourse of breast disease is constructed in terms of individuals who are at high risk for genetic reasons, like Eastern European jews, or lifestyle issues like smoking or eating too much fat. Environmental devastation and hazards are most often silenced, and with them their racial and class aspects are smothered as well. Pesticides and industrial pollutants are treated as inevitable, and naturalized as part of our landscape as such. There is faint recognition that poorer people, living in areas closer to industry and its pollution, suffer these consequences more directly.

The racial component of this economic inequality is ignored while women of color with breast cancer are largely excluded—inadvertently or not—from drug trials. A woman first needs to have access to the information about a trial before she can enter it. In order to participate in a trial, a woman needs to be able to take time off from work as well as have the means to travel to the trial's facility. She needs health insurance to help defray the costs involved, and so on. Many managed care companies will not cover participation in any kind of drug trial. These social and economic networks bespeak class and racial location.

Corporate economic self-interest sets too much of the context for breast cancer. It infects breast cancer protocols and their presentation of information. Breast Cancer Awareness Month (BCAM) is a disturbing example of how the political economy orchestrates and narrows women's access to information. BCAM is sponsored by the Zeneca pharmaceutical firm that manufactures Nolvadex, better known as tamoxifen. Tamoxifen is now marketed, as "the best prevention for breast cancer," along with mammography. Meanwhile tamoxifen brings in $470 million a year for Zeneca, while Zeneca also produces acetochlor, a cancer-causing chlorine-based herbicide.[9]

The message of BCAM is that the best prevention is early detection. But detection is *not* prevention. As well, careful skepticism must be used about embracing cancer drugs that are manufactured by the very same companies that produce the toxins and carcinogenic chemicals that can initiate and instigate malignancies in the first place. I will return here.

Over thirty years ago the World Health Organization concluded that

80 percent of cancers were due to "human produced carcinogens." Over 73 twenty years ago the National Institutes of Health identified environmental factors as the major cause of most cancers.[10] Yet it is repeatedly said that we do not know what causes breast cancer, while a notion of it as genetically inherited remains center stage.

Genetic familial breast cancer calls forth an image of static and unchangeable genes, determining one's life. This autonomous and ahistorical viewing of genes reflects a corporeal and physiological abstractness that disconnects bodies from their cultural and economic moorings. I see bodies as partly genetic and genetics as partly tendencies or proclivities awaiting their environments.[11]

This abstracted corporeality, disconnected from the multiple environs defining it, also affects the prevalent discussions of estrogen as hormonally driving breast cancer. It is widely accepted that estrogen causes breast cells, and cells of other reproductive organs, to divide and grow.[12] Protocols for treatment, like the use of tamoxifen as an antiestrogen, follow from this hormonal stance.

I am hesitant to accept the dominance of the estrogen narrative. Although some breast cancers are instigated by estrogen levels, others are not. Although estrogen is thought to play a significant role in cell division, the thought is less rigorous than presented. Very little is really understood about the part estrogen plays, and with what specific effects.

There are multiple and various sources of estrogen both inside and outside the body. Therefore, there is no static, universal, pregiven amount of estrogen in any one woman's body. One's estrogen level will vary according to one's unique ovaries and their environments. And hormonal status changes over time. The knowable and specified amount of estrogen will differ from one woman's body to another.

Discussion of estrogen based breast cancer assumes an exactitude of knowledge that does not exist. I know no one who has tried estrogen replacement therapy who believes that her doctor knew the amounts necessary for her before the process of trial and error began. It very often takes months to figure the dosage out, and sometimes it cannot be found.

Much of the estrogen narrative distorts what is known about breast

74 cancer. At best, it is just a very partial viewing of a much larger and more complex problem. Estrogen receptors are found in about 65 to 80 percent of breast cancers in postmenopausal women; and in 45 to 60 percent of breast cancers in premenopausal women.[13] What about the 35 to 55 percent of women with non-estrogen-receptor breast cancer? A larger scoping of the disease is needed.

The depictions of breast cancer as either familial or estrogen driven are partial and incomplete. At its best this viewing inappropriately disguises itself as scientific. It decontextualizes and dehistoricizes breast cancer instead of searching to contextualize the relationship between various estrogen levels, genetic makeup, and the impact on them of their multiple environments. In part this means that women's bodies need to be specified by the local environments that they inhabit within their larger global context. I am writing not of some oversimplified causal relation that reduces all to the environs, but rather of a complex and changing set of relationships between breast tissue and the influences on it.

The extremes between wealth and poverty continue to increase, around the world and in the u.s. There is less protection of the environment, less protection in the workplace, less protection of the air and water and soil. During the Reagan-Bush-Clinton decades public health has been jeopardized by increasing privatization. In the u.s., public health is undermined by less federal regulation of workplaces. Imported foods have little if any restrictions on the use of toxins. There is less labeling of foodstuffs containing harmful additives or derived from biochemical processes and genetically altered crops. Food contamination arises more frequently. This contributes to environments that undermine the health of our bodies leaving them, more vulnerable to genetic mutations.

The dominant breast cancer discourses smother the complexity of the multifactors at play. Much of the scientific literature and research is focused on a single cause. It is either diet, or environmental carcinogens, or radiation, or genes, or fat, or estrogen that causes breast cancer. But even the few breast cancers that are biogenetic are still probably triggered by their environments. The borders of the breast, and the

body, and even their genes are multiple and changing. As such the economic, and racial, and cultural inequality of these environments is a
part of the body itself. Nancy Krieger says that discrimination and inequality are reflected in and on our bodies. Our bodies are not just biological. They are simultaneously economic and social and cultural.
Then biology itself can become discriminatory.[14]

Much of the cancer establishment—the drug industry, pharmaceutical companies, government health agencies, the American Medical
Association (AMA), research labs, and cancer foundations—obfuscates
what is truly known about breast cancer by authorizing partial medical
and scientific findings as something more. Global capital's investment
in portions of the cancer establishment does not assist in making a critique of the very structures that underpin its empire. This is no simple
case of dishonesty or lying or conspiracy. It rather reflects the complicated and compromised relations between the labs, funding agencies,
established cancer foundations, and drug companies that set the so-
called scientific agendas.

New narratives are needed to dislodge the naturalized assumptions
of mainstream medicine.[15] Women's corporeality is open and fluid. The
parallel to global capital, which smashes national economic borders, is
significant. The contaminated air of the Chernobyl nuclear disaster, the
bombings and resulting pollution over iraq and kosovo, the oil spills into
our global waterways filter across the boundaries of the air we breathe
and maybe the estrogen we produce.

Science is a part of the larger cultural and political landscape and
reflects and constructs the social forces of which it is a part. Scientific
knowledge, regardless of its claims to objectivity, is not structured differently from any other knowledge base. Breast cancer research, drug trials,
and so on are "distinctive social products which are constituted and actualized in social practice."[16]

There is a curious conundrum here. While any and every cancer researcher would love to discover a cure, there are also political and economic dynamics that work against this. Although global capital is
incredibly antidemocratic (the rich are getting richer and the poor are
getting poorer), cancer is somewhat more democratic in that anyone

76 can develop it. Rich *and* poor die from breast cancer, although their access to detection and treatments will vary greatly, as well as their exposure to carcinogens. My point is not that capitalism, or its environs, alone causes breast cancer. Instead, its antiecological consumerist priorities define a particular historical setting that invades and makes multirelational viewing impossible. The science we need is squashed by this capitalist, masculinist, and racialized frame of reference that naturalizes and neutralizes ecological and bodily devastation.

In this sense, breast cancer is truly manmade.

## Reconstructing Breast Cancer

Let me reimagine the breast. Connect it to the body systemically and to its complex environments cyclically. Define our environments with open yet connected boundaries between air, water, soil, economic and racial hierarchies, and the female body.

Interrogate the cause/effect scientific model for its linear blinders. Supplant this model with an interactive and multistage model of malignant growth that recognizes the interstices between bodies, genes, and environments. Such an *epistēmē* will need to critically address the conflicting messages about women's bodies, their socially and environmentally constructed genes, and the role of genes in breast cancer.

Cancer is then to be seen as a multifactorial, multimechanistic, multistaged process. A once regular cell has lost its brakes and is growing out of control. Cancer cells are promoted and initiated by damage to the cell's genetic material, to which some genetic material is more vulnerable than others. Very often exposure takes years to metabolize. There can be multiple origins and a complicated set of elusive and ambiguous assaults before cells succumb to malignancy. Relationships, contextuality, and coincidence need to be recognized as part of this process.

A systemic starting point that sees the body as part of the environment with fluid boundaries necessitates a multipurpose orientation. The breasts are distinct but not separate from the body; the body is distinct but not separate from the air it breathes and water it drinks. And if we draw from Nawal El Saadawi's view that one's health involves all

one's body parts including the mind, then the cultural environment that   77
fetishizes breasts and nourishes anxiety, perhaps contributing to delay in
treatment, or denial, plays an important role here too.[17]

As Sandra Steingraber says so poignantly: "A cancer cell, then, is
made, not born." Cancer arises from a series of incremental changes to
chromosomal DNA, and the changes are instigated environmentally.
Cancer runs in her family—but her family is adopted, not biological.
Families share both chromosomes *and* environments. "What runs in
families does not necessarily run in blood."[18]

The chromosomal body is already imbricated in its environs and
surroundings. This is not to say that the biological health of the body
does not have a status to reckon with. I have experienced my body too
many ways not to know this. But its biogenetic autonomy, whatever this
means, is also compromised by environmental pesticides, herbicides,
and manmade ideological preferences about women's bodies.

A static biologized and racialized viewing of genes is more political
than it is scientific. It is a view that often finds validity in politically reac-
tionary times. There is little surprise that it has a renewed appeal for the
twenty-first century of global capital. The privatized discourse of neoliberalism makes the individual responsible for his or her condition
whether that be poverty or illness.

Individuals are said to be what they make of themselves; they are
supposed to work hard to make the most of their biological inheritance.
Health becomes a sign of individual discipline: one exercises sufficiently, does not eat too much fat, takes the necessary dietary supplements, and so on. This fuels the self-help health industry, which tells us
we can heal ourselves. This privatized view of health assumes independent rather than interrelated selves defined by one's life choices and experiences. Such independent autonomy always assumes the wealth
necessary to be self-sufficient. And inequality and discrimination are
once again silenced in this scenario.

My daughter's high school health class adopts this individualized
view of health. It is up to these girls to be healthy: do not smoke or
drink, eat low fat, and so on. The course's definition of high risk is determined by your familial history. So it is up to Sarah to be healthy on the

78   one hand, although it is also assumed that she won't be healthy, given her genetic trajectory. I wish Sarah's health course helped teenage girls work at being healthy *and* also made clear the larger environmental framing of breast disease. And I wish that genetics would be viewed as a disposition that may or may not actualize.

For many women today, cancer seems as inevitable as global capital. However, whereas the cancer is feared and despised, the latter is embraced. Yet environmental destruction by global capital may make the destructiveness of biogenetics unstoppable. One-half of all cancers are in the industrialized world, although only one-fifth of the population is located here.[19] This attitude of inevitability destroys the potential for a new visibility.

Breast cancer can be used as an opening up of the interior body to its exterior dimensions. In this way I view breast cancer as an "interiorization of the outside," "an interior of the exterior," where we can see the hierarchical relations of class and racialized gender inside/out of the body.[20] The Women's Community Cancer Project in Boston speaks similarly in its "Women Cancer Agenda." Breast cancer is reframed here as a social and political/biological problem defined by the food and tobacco industry, the military-industrial complex, and corporate polluters. The Agenda calls for research that recognizes the interdependence of the whole individual in her social and political context, not just the cancer cells in her body.[21]

The war against cancer has been likened to a "medical Vietnam."[22] Although it is estimated that as much as 80 percent of cancers may be avoidable and preventable, cancer continues to increase at the rate of 1 percent a year since 1950 in the u.s., canada, japan, and denmark.[23]

While women across the globe struggle for peace in bosnia, pakistan, and algeria, and lead the movements to save environments in Africa, women in the u.s. are offered tamoxifen and testing for the BRCA1 and 2 genes if they are considered at high risk. These offerings are not helpful enough for any of us. Instead, women must demand that science and the cancer industry begin to think like a mountain, or a river.[24] This means viewing environments as rhizomed with the body at multiple complexly webbed locations.

Breast health demands a rethinking of the politics of the body and
the body of politics. This demands an unsilencing of the naturalized
starting places of an already politicized science. Singular causality is
challenged. In its place knots of multiplicity and fluidity allow us to en-
tertain the difference between really knowing, maybe knowing, and not
knowing. This is a healthier starting place for the breast.

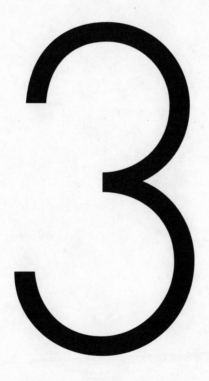

# 3

Politicizing Personal
Environments

# Pluralized Environments in Black and White

SARAH AND GIAH TOOK THE BIRTH CONTROL PILL. Sarah used it for over a decade; Giah a few years less. I so often wonder whether the pill disrupted the delicate integrity of their bodies and unleashed their genetic disposition toward breast cancer. I sometimes think that they would not have succumbed to cancerous gene mutations if they had not taken the pill. Sometimes I think that breast cancer was written through their genes no matter what. Other times I wonder if their cancers would have developed later in their lives without the pill. Less frequently, I try to figure out the other exposures that compromised their bodies and later mine.

It is strange how often the old construct of nature/culture reappears. I cyclically and repetitively return to this issue over and over again. Which matters more—the body or its surroundings? Sex or gender? Genetics or race? How much does each really impact on the other? These queries are hardly new.

84     Do bodies have their own genetic determination, or do environments matter as much, or more, or at all? I speak of environment in the plural because it is not a singular space or identity for me. Environments contain a series of what I see as rhizomed knots that often cannot be unraveled into singular sites, although sometimes they can be.

The environment, as a singular location, is often envisioned as the outer, natural layering of air, water, and soil that is later undermined by manmade pollutants. The body is seen as a separate entity whose identity can then be environmentally compromised. But the very notion of an inside (body) and outside (environs) distorts the real complexity of the relationship. As Sharon Thomson of the Community Arts and Education Project says: "What is happening to our earth is happening to our breasts."[1] My project recognizes the interpenetration of bodies and their overlapping environments.

Bodies have genetic dispositions and potentials but are not simply determined either biologically or environmentally. I respect and fear both the biological and the environmental—both for their independent effect and their intertwining overlap. Even the few breast cancers that are biogenetically inherited are still probably triggered by their environments. Cell mutation is a long-term process.

## Seeing Plural Environments

My notion of environments includes the knotted layerings that are unnatural, that are manmade, that construct the disregard for clean air, or fresh water, or healthy bodies. Environments and diseases alike are socially constructed, although they also always contain remnants of what I hesitantly call their biogenetic potential. You know that air is polluted because there is an idea of nonpolluted air. You know a diseased cell, because there is such a thing as a healthy cell. This relational meaning creates a vital tension between what exists and what might exist, what has been created and what might be created.

Our environs simultaneously contain the effects of the relations of power and also the possibility of different arrangements. I see racism,

and sexism, and class privilege as already encrusted onto and into our    85
physical bodies and surroundings. There is very little that is natural or
given. When these politicized layerings are neutralized as part of the
naturalized landscape, no one asks why more black and latino women
are not part of breast cancer drug trials, or why Viagra was not developed first for women, or why silicon breast implants were ever marketed
in the first place. Silence these initial queries and we are already in polluted waters.

I am not proposing some kind of environmentalist reductionism that
collapses effects to a singular environmental factor working in isolation.
Nor am I saying that the environments we inhabit capture the entirety
of the problem. Nor do I mean to imply that if we focus on the environs
of the body, everything will be changeable or preventable. Actually, I
sometimes think it might be easier to change the body than the power
structures that dominate in our environments. Yet Sarah's and Giah's
deaths have left scars that are too deep. Even if the environs of poverty,
racism, masculinism, the workforce, are radically changed, some bodies
will succumb to their mutated cells.

The distinctness—of the body and its outside surroundings—is both
real and not real. Environments do not simply surround but also perme-
ate, and the environs are affected and altered by human invention. Environments encircle *and* are invasive. It is more than suggestive that
women in Africa and Asia have so much less breast cancer. Their long-
term dietary patterns are primarily plant based. They eat whole grains
and cereals that are not processed.[2] But I am also sure that there is no
one single factor operating here.

One's nutritional environment—defined by both culture and local
agriculture—appears to matter in some degree. The globalizing of the
economy may change all this soon enough. But for now a plant- rather
than an animal-based diet affects cancer rates, even though this is only
one factor in a multifactorial disease process.

I argue that breast cancer is more socially, economically, and racially
constructed than it is genetically inherited. This means understanding a
range of social factors: an increased number of women being exposed to

86  toxicity in the workplace, shifting discourses about women's health, so-
called science narratives with their masculinist and racialized assumptions, and global capital with its petro/chemical-pharmaceutical empire
and postindustrial-medical complex.

These plural environments set the context of breast health. The environments of nature, of the political economy, of culture, of racism and
sexism intersect with each other, creating devastating combinations.
These environments are defined in and through complex systems of
power like the postindustrial-medical complex, the petro/chemical-
pharmaceutical/cosmetic complex, the cyber/media-corporate complex.
I wish there were less cumbersome ways to call attention to these complexes of power but I have not found them. Because corporate priorities
construct the global agenda, these complexes overlap with each other to
articulate and popularize the public's understanding of breast health.
Progressive health movements find themselves poised with and against
these powerful forces.

Environments are both sites and locations *and* the set of power relations that define them. These environments that nurture breast cancer
tissue are more formidable for almost all women than genetic proclivity.
This view is controversial because it undermines the staticized and nat-
uralized/biogenetic standpoint as a nonneutral starting place.

The environs of masculinist culture, which fantasizes the breast as a
floating symbol of womanhood often disconnected from head and torso,
psychically operates to disconnect breast cancer from its environmental
moorings along with its body. This master fantasy of female beauty is
singularly of white women's breasts. These masculinist visions get smug-
gled into and out of the domains of the postindustrial-medical and
petro/chemical-pharmaceutical/cosmetic corporate complexes. They
then leech into medical research, treatment, prevention, and even some
kinds of advocacy.

My *epistēmē* is not wholly satisfying. Environments matter, but they
do not erase the significance of the actual body or its breast tissue. Genetic dispositions are very often declarative and yet different stories
unfold from them. This is a complicated mixing of inside in the outside;

genetic in the societal; individual in the racialized gender structures;   87
and personal in the political. The intertwining recombines each side of
the divide, leaving neither side the same as it was, yet neither equivalent
with the other. The divide exists and does not.

Environmental hazards enter breast tissue, stay there, and change
the health of the breast. And the breast is part of the body, so the entire
system of the body attempts to adjust to these assaults. However, mutated breast genes do not affect the environment. Genes are not hazardous to others in the environs in the way petro/chemical pollutants
may be. Breast cancer genes have little public effect; just the misery of
private mourning. A method that keeps its eye on the political and cultural and economic racial structuring of environments should have
clear priority when considering the public health.

## The Environmentalist's Environment

When the term "environment" is used in its popularized form, it is
visioned as a natural habitat that needs protection. It is used to elicit the
idea of a natural, untouched, and pure state of things. This image is
contrasted with the interventions and misuse of corporate projects. En-
vironmentalism, as a critically activist stance against the exploitation of
the globe's natural resources, privileges the cycles of nature and demands their protection. Nature's habitat—soil, air, insects, and water—
have their own life cycles and requisites that need preservation.

Environmentalists condemn the abuse of the natural order. Air is
polluted as a result of the Gulf War in iraq, pesticides are routinely used
in housing projects in the u.s., poor rural communities in the u.s. find
themselves awash in waste dump sites, agribusiness contaminates the
soil in mexico, and so on. A form of environmental racism emerges that
harms poor people of color the most directly.

Environmental racism is a form of discrimination that expresses
both economic class and white/anglo racial privilege. Laws and zoning
codes are enforced in racially and economically discriminatory ways.
Poor communities disproportionately populated by people of color are

88    the most directly affected by waste landfills, chemical factories, lead smelters, and so on. In Los Angeles County 90 percent of the waste-producing facilities are located in minority communities.[3]

People's bodies absorb their environments, so there are particular consequences to where we live. Yet air and water also drift and seep across national boundaries and disperse the damage beyond one's local habitat. The Chernobyl nuclear disaster makes clear that a local event has consequences far beyond its initial location. Anna Volchkova lives in belarus, where 70 percent of the area was directly contaminated from Chernobyl. Her entire family is sick, and her youngest son, who was born after the accident, suffers from poor digestion and motor skills. His entire nervous system has been affected. "All the children have lowered immunity and need constant rest. No one laughs anymore."[4]

Depleted uranium was used as a cheap coating for the bombs dropped during the Gulf War. DU, a form of nuclear waste, produces a fine dust when burnt that enters the food chain. Cancers have risen tenfold in iraq since 1991.[5] Mayor Giuliani of New York City along with the Centers for Disease Control authorized the spraying of malathion, declaring it as only slightly toxic, over parts of New York to combat the West Nile Virus. However, the label on malathion reads: "Do not apply this product in a way that will contact workers or other persons either directly or through drift."[6] Thus this attempt to address people's health concerns creates a heartbreaking challenge for people's health.

It is crucial to try and preserve, as best we can, what is left of the natural habitat even though enormously powerful forces vie against us. These nexuses of power—the postindustrial-medical complex, the petro/chemical-pharmaceutical/cosmetic complex, and the cyber/media corporate complex—overlap and knot together in formidable ways.

This complicated knotted rhizome of power constructs a transnational corporate hierarchy of global capital. This corporate complex of power is not, however, a unified whole. Internal conflicts arise from competing needs within its constituent parts. Corporate locations of power shift as global capital continually renegotiates its relation to nation states. With as much as 17 percent of the u.s. economy tied to

medical services and pharmaceutical products, corporatized medical    89
science takes on a new significance. As a trans-nation-state apparatus
evolves, the cancer establishment vies for a privileged location within it.

There would be a wildly different political agenda if the public
health were the key concern. Agricultural pesticides would be largely
eliminated. Foods would not be packaged in carcinogenic plastics.
Cows would not be injected with hormones such as rbST to increase
milk production. Instead, the stock market guides those in the seats of
power. These types of choices are not part of a natural landscape but
rather are specifically derivative of a corporate-consumer mentality set
on efficiency, productivity, and profitability. This mental set draws the
parameters for a particular kind of science. It makes it harder to get
grant money for interdisciplinary research, which attempts to look at the
multiple factors defining chemical risk.

Carlos Sonnenschein and Ana Soto in their lab at Tufts University
found that the plastic tubing they were using in their experiments
caused "rampant proliferation" of breast cancer cells. They found plastics to be "biologically active," acting like hormone mimickers.[7] There
are now several more scientists who believe plastics act like estrogen
mimics and disrupt normal hormone function. This is enough for me to
say that plastics are too dangerous to the public health to have them in
use.

There are approximately three hundred manmade chemicals that
have been identified as cancer causing by the National Toxicology Program of the Environmental Protection Agency. Yet herbicide and pesticide use continues. Although DDT (dichloro-diphenyl-trichloro-
ethane) was banned in the u.s. in 1972, it remains in use as a cheap and
effective control for malaria in most poor countries. As late as 1991, the
u.s. exported at least 4.1 million pounds of pesticides banned or suspended from use here, including 96 tons of DDT.[8]

In 1995, $234 billion worth of chemical products were sold by the
one hundred largest chemical manufacturers.[9] Five billion pounds of
pesticides were used in 1989, which included sixteen hundred different
chemicals. Thirty times more pesticides were used in the u.s. in 1990

90 than in 1945.[10] Given the multiple exposures to several chemicals at any
one time, it is almost impossible to attribute singular causality to any
one chemical.

Toxic solvents, solid-waste landfill gases, and assorted petrochemicals are also recognized by a minority of scientists to compromise the
immune system. Many carcinogens like benzopyrene act as immuno-
suppressants. Formaldehyde (used in veneers) and perchloroethylene
(dry cleaning solvent) are highly suspect as carcinogenic. Workplace
chemicals and chemicals in the plastics industry are thought to be similarly harmful.[11]

The priorities of the public health cannot be set by the very companies benefiting from the sale of these petrochemicals. It is dangerous to
continue the further contamination of the earth, air, and waterways
without rethinking where this is taking most of the people across the
globe. The effects are devastating for the public health and the personal
health of even the profiteers.

The privatized health care system in the u.s., where more than forty
million people do not have the insurance that allows them access to
care, becomes a further detrimental part of this environmental system.
Profit making from the sale of harmful chemicals is acceptable in this
nexus of global capital, and so is the privatized and limited health care
that emerges from the same agenda. Lack of commitment to the public
health—in terms of either prevention of disease or its treatment—ruins
many personal lives. The medical industry services fewer and fewer people, while the petrochemical industries undermine the health of more
and more.

The health of the breast cannot be sufficiently addressed from
within this politicized environment. Andrea Martin, founder of the
Breast Cancer Fund in San Francisco, is committed to revealing this
connection between breast cancer and its environment. The Fund believes that toxic and synthetic chemicals, plastics, detergents, and pesticides grow cancer cells. It believes this focus should be central to breast
cancer activists.[12]

*Rachel's Environment*

Rachel Carson testified before Congress in 1963 about the harmful effects of pesticide use. Pesticides were killing birds in Duxbury, Massachusetts. Her work led to a ban on the insecticide DDT. But much else related to her concern with the overall harmful long-term effects of pesticides on the natural cycles that exist between insects, air, water, and soil has been ignored.

Pesticides are supposed to kill "pests": insects, weeds, and rodents. These synthetic chemicals contaminate streams and groundwater and enter the bodies of fish and birds. They have "enormous biological potency" and destroy the enzymes whose function it is to protect the body. Without the proper oxidation from which the body gets energy, some cells will start on the road to malignancy.[13]

Spray dusts are used to protect farm crops, aerosol disinfectants are used in homes to kill bugs, weed killers are regularly used in gardens. These practices contaminate and alter the tissues of plants and animals and can alter hereditary lineage.[14] These are all processes that are not visible to the naked eye and therefore are easy to ignore.

For Carson, much of pest control negates needed "natural cycles." Some birds depend on insects for their food. When the insects are killed, the entire cycle shifts. She was concerned with the way pesticides interact with each other to form deadly combinations. The effects on the synergy between humans, plants, and animals are multiple. DDT kills indiscriminately and harmfully intervenes in this complex network of relations.

Carson's viewing of the environment requires that one recognize that harm cannot always be seen, that it is most probably a result of multiple chemicals interacting in combination with one another, and that it develops slowly over time. Contaminated water and air most often do not smell. An individual chemical may not be harmful when ingested by itself but becomes toxic in interaction with other pesticides. This way of thinking requires a vision of an interacting system of relations that are

92  interdependent and historically linked. It requires an *epistēmē* that sees the unseeable, thinks in multiplicity, and over long periods of time. A similar view needs to be extended to the nutritional understanding of people's bodies.

POPS (Persistent Organic Pollutants) are named for their long-term persistence in the environment, long after their use is over. They resist being broken down by sunlight. They are fat soluble so they concentrate and move up the food chain. An intergovernmental negotiation committee, made up of governments from more than 150 countries, is attempting to draw up a binding global treaty demanding the reduction and/or elimination of twelve of these toxic chemicals worldwide. A much-used chemical, dioxin, heads the list.[15]

Although toxic pesticides and industrial pollutants are recognized as global poisons, they continue to be used across much of the poorest parts of the globe. These toxins remain hazardous at all points of their life cycle: manufacture, transportation, and final disposal.

Noted ecologist Sandra Steingraber argues that the leading carcinogen, dioxin, is thought to inhabit the tissues of every living person, as well as the breast milk of women. She describes the pesticide and industrial chemical contamination of the groundwater and surface waters of central Illinois. She draws critical attention to the insidious presence of contaminants in our lives like vinyl chloride, which is thought to be as dangerous as dioxin. The vinyl is used to make credit cards, garden hoses, lawn furniture, and food packaging, each of which have become a regular part of daily life.[16]

Environmental carcinogens and pesticide residues have large-scale unintended consequences. They end up in unexpected places including the food we eat and water we drink. Water, used to wash fruits and vegetables or irrigate the soil, if it contains traces of weed killer or dry cleaning fluid, can promote cancer creating pathways to people's bodies. Once one recognizes the reproducibility of contamination via multiple sites—especially via air, water, and soil—the impact and effects of dangerous herbicides and pesticides become much more urgent. Our thinking must look for, and uncover, this knotted rhizomed complexity.

Given the intransigency of global priorities and what feels like in- credibly limited political alternatives, many people, including myself, opt for at least trying to protect our own bodies as best we can. But these attempts at health are individualized and privatized. Those privileged enough to do so buy natural foods, bottled water, nutrients, and so forth. To the extent that environments are already inside our bodies, this personalized approach is obviously inadequate.

## Changing the Body's Environs

I hope that by controlling and changing my diet and my daughter's, we can fool the process of mutation. I try in every way I know to see that she stays healthy. I hope I can change my body—as a host environment—enough that cancer cells won't replicate again. I fantasize that if there are cells, they will just stay dormant. But I also know the limits of all this.

Even if one can afford to buy organic produce, there is no guarantee that this produce is not unintentionally affected by soil or water that is already contaminated. Recognizing the large-scale corporate impact on bodily health focuses attention on the structural constraints within which our individual health choices exist. It is too easy to think that we have control over our health because of the vast consumer market of nutrients, vitamins, immune system boosters, and so on. But it is also the case that the organic food industry and vitamin/nutrient companies operate within a market-driven economy, the same economy that destroys the vitamin content of food to begin with. Alongside the billion-dollar food supplement industry exists a food industry that ignores issues of pesticide harm, uses processing techniques that destroy vitamin content, develops fat-free foods with known undesirable side effects.[17]

Diet, particularly in relation to breast cancer, is big business today. Newsweek's cover story in late 1998 was "Cancer and Diet." The subtitle read: "Eating to Beat the Odds." We are told to use olive oil and flaxseed; wheat bran and whole grains; fruits and dark green leafy vegetables; salmon and garlic.[18] Jane Brody of the New York Times states in

94   her "Personal Health" column that diet, although not a panacea, cuts
the risk of cancer. Grains like wheat, rice, corn, barley, oats, and rye are
recommended.[19]

Mortality rates from breast cancer in china are five times lower than
in the u.s. In china, 70 percent of a woman's calories come from carbo-
hydrates, compared with 40 percent in the u.s. In the u.s. 70 percent or
more of protein comes from animal foods; in china, 7 percent does, with
93 percent coming from plant and grain sources.[20] Soy is thought to
work possibly as an antiestrogen, competing with the body's estrogen,
binding to receptors.

Nutrition is emerging in sectors of breast cancer discourse as a very
important method of prevention, and I follow just about all the recom-
mendations stated above.[21] But most of the diet talk does not query the
healthy status of the foods we eat. One could assume that nonorganic
strawberries are healthy to eat because they are a fruit. But one also
needs to know that strawberries have an incredibly high pesticide usage.
Information is too often partial and incomplete.

Nevertheless, if one's health is a long-term process, it is important to
do as much as one can individually and personally to limit the larger societal impact, whether that be pesticide use, food carcinogens, or environmental racism.

Too many people do not earn enough today to be able to spend
money trying to stay healthy. If your job is located in a contaminated
area, there is too often little you can do to change it. Too many people
do not have health insurance. Nutritional supplements are not covered
on most health plans. Organic food costs significantly more than nonorganic. Health-food stores with organic produce do not exist in many
communities.

The disregard for the earth's health emanates from the priorities of
global capital, which disregards the collective realities of people across
the globe. This does not mean that cancer is simply caused by global
capital and is completely new. There is evidence of cancerous tumors in
dinosaur bones and the human tissue of egyptian mummies.[22] But cancer is affecting more and more people. The effects of global capital —
poverty for great numbers, air pollution and soil depletion — create

environments that are disproportionately cancer producing, especially
for poor people of color.

## Environmental Racism and Female Bodies

Many of the environmental justice groups in San Diego, Tijuana, and Detroit are made up of low-income people of color who first started fighting toxic contamination in their own neighborhoods.[23] Similarly, environmental protection is becoming a major concern of third-world countries of the south and east in Africa and india. The exploitation of these countries is part and parcel of the destruction of their natural environments. Some 99 percent of india's original forest has been lost, while 57 percent of its current forest remains threatened.[24]

The globalization of capital in agriculture and agrifood systems has increased the levels of pesticide use and therefore the contamination of food.[25] Since the 1950s new synthetic fertilizers have been used to replace the natural fertility of the soil, which has been depleted by overuse.[26] The maximization of profits, not the concerns with the hungry, underlies the overuse of soil. As such, capitalistic notions of efficiency define an economic set of choices that strains the ecosystem with excessive use and synthetic products.[27]

This view of capital's disregard for the earth's resources contextualizes environmental concerns. The problem is not one of the environment per se. The problem derives from capital's presumption that the natural environment—land, trees, oil, minerals, water—is exploitable and renewable. Bodily health is not viewed as integral to its environs. My hypothesis of a porous genetic body that absorbs environmental processes over time requires a humanized standpoint that recognizes the racialized and class aspects of these processes.

An eighty-five-mile stretch along the Mississippi River between New Orleans and Baton Rouge is home to over 140 petrochemical and other industrial plants. Convent, Louisiana, which is located here, is predominantly poor and african-american. Each year, Shintech, the main chemical corporation housed here, produces 1.1 billion pounds of polyvinyl chloride (PVC). Shintech emits almost three hundred pounds of indus-

96   trial poisons for each individual in Convent each year. In this heart of what has come to be called "cancer alley," the level of toxicity is sky high.[28]

Why is it that cancer mortality rates are higher for blacks than for whites? Why is it that the air is filthier in these black communities? Environmental toxins increase according to poverty, and disproportionate numbers of blacks are poor. These communities have less access to medical diagnosis and treatment. Women covered by medicaid were more than two times more likely than privately insured women to be diagnosed with late-stage disease.[29] Thus race, class, and health hazards combine. Meanwhile, most breast cancer drug trials are of white middle-class women. Yet the so-called scientific talk of breast cancer assumes it is shared alike by women.

Too much is unknown here. Because black women are silenced within the racialized discourses of white femininity, fantasized female beauty presumes white breasts. Black women's breasts, like their bodies, are encoded by these racialized meanings. This silencing and marginalizing by racialized environments overlap with black women's lesser access to preventive medical care and their later detection of breast cancer.

Women in the San Francisco Bay Area have the highest rates of breast cancer of any women living in western countries. According to Mary Anglin, african-american women in the Bay Area have the fourth-highest rate of breast cancer in the world. They, as well as most poor women, have to fight the Departments of Social Services and Health Departments in order to get mammograms. They often are put on waiting lists for six to nine months. These same women have little access to experimental therapies and clinical trials or to major medical centers and research facilities. Although the trials themselves do not cost money, the follow-up care does. Women without health insurance, or with insurance that does not pay for experimental procedures, have to have their own independent means.[30]

This may in part explain why, although there is a higher incidence rate of breast cancer among white women, black women have a higher mortality rate.[31] Nancy Krieger specifies differentials of survival along

racial and class lines. Working-class and poor women, who are dispro- 97
portionately black and latino, live fewer years than professional and affluent women, who are more often white. Racial disparities in
socioeconomic position suggest a link between one's class and one's survival. It is also often the case that working-class women are more likely
than affluent women to be already suffering from other adverse health
conditions, like diabetes or heart disease. The meaning of race itself becomes multifactorial.

Late-stage diagnosis and lack of medical access, an intimate part of
the politics of racism, define the varied realities of breast cancer.[32]
Krieger digs deeply into the comparisons between black and white
women across class lines. She finds that the incidence rates of black and
white women differ in part according to age. For women over forty, the
breast cancer rate is higher among white women. But for women under
the age of forty, rates are higher among black women. She queries the
difference and wonders about the significance of adolescence in this
process as well as the use of oral contraceptives and abortion. White
women, with a higher class standing, have a later age for first full-term
pregnancy and an earlier age of menarche. But there are few readily
available explanations for these variations.

Krieger finds the greatest risk for black women is for those under
forty living in professional homes; whereas the greatest risk for white
women is for those over forty living in working-class homes. Class and
race play a part here: young black women are at greater risk the wealth-
ier they are. The association between decreasing age at menarche and
higher risk for middle-class and educated whites does not hold for young
black women.[33] An environment of racially coded class experience appears as an element in this particular narration of breast cancer, but the
complex relations are still not self-evident.

We are left to further examine how pregnancy and age of menarche—relating to amounts of estrogen exposure—cross over racial and
class lines. But we need to be careful how we think of estrogen; to include both its endogenous and exogenous forms. Estrogen level then
may be as important in environmental racism as it is in female ovaries.

The relationship between race and racism and their complex

98  connection with economic class are crucial for a better understanding of black women's breast cancer. Zora Brown of the Breast Cancer Resource Committee in Washington worries that "black women in general are facing a more aggressive form of the disease." Black women are "fifty percent more likely than white women to get breast cancer before the age of 35 and they are 50 percent more likely to die of it before they turn fifty." Some of this disparity is identified with inequalities of access to diagnosis and good follow-up care. But others are wondering whether black women's breast cancer is in part reflective of a different tumor biology, one that is less estrogen-receptor based. As Ngina Lythcott of the Mailman Columbia University School of Public Health says, "When black women get together and talk about their tremendous fear of getting breast cancer, the fear is that it's a disease that's different from other breast cancer." Brown reiterates this concern when she says that "we need to do very focused research on African-American women and breast cancer."[34] Absolutely we do.

Such research needs to embrace a multifactored complex nodal approach that recognizes the intersections between race and class within black women's environments. This approach does not necessarily reject the possibility that there is a specific biogenetic dimension to black women's breast cancer but rather demands the contextualization of this dimension. If black women seem more prone to non-estrogen-dependent tumors, then comparisons are needed between this population and the significant group of white women whose tumors are also non–estrogen dependent. Whatever the biogenetic racial story is, it is also always imbricated in the larger system of racism with its economic effects.

So if there is a racial biogenetics of breast cancer to discover, it is never singularly that. Genetic mutations are dispositions awaiting triggers. And the triggers may be as significant as, or more significant than, the genetic site itself. We should be very cautious not to overstate the determinacy of genetic markings. The sedimented layers of racism with their discriminatory economic impact must be theorized into any breast cancer racial genetic coding. The choices here are not biologic race or class or environments because the overlapping relations of poverty, diet, contaminated environs, and so on feed on each other.

Biogenetic race is more often used as a mask for racism than as a

starting point for unpacking the multiplicity of disease formation. This is    99
not to negate any particular biogenetic explanation but rather to redirect
the evaluation of what biogenetic complexly means.

When I met with Ngina Lythcott at the Mailman School, I first
asked her if she thought there was a breast cancer unique to black
women. She said there may be for some black women, but that we have
not done the research to know much of anything yet. She also believes
that racism is an environmental risk for all black women, middle class
and poor alike. "Discrimination is toxic for us all, even if we experience
it at different levels of intensity." Lythcott, the daughter of medical doctors, still grew up in segregated neighborhoods. She movingly and halt-
ingly says that if you are black, no matter what your class is, "living as
the 'other' creates chronic tension and forces you to live protecting your-
self from the next psychic wound." The "constant vigilance" takes its
toll, on top of the other rigors of daily life.[35]

Lythcott had several important ideas about how to redirect and devise methods for addressing black women's issues. She stressed the need
for connecting the science done in the lab to primary care physicians;
developing grassroots medical care more consistently; building research
facilities and funding for researchers of color; funding research done in
women of color communities; and focusing more on population-based
science rather on than lab science. She readily agreed with my sugges-
tions to devise comparative studies between african-american women
and ashkenazi jews with the BRCA1 and 2 gene. And we both thought
controlled studies comparing u.s. black women with African blacks
would also reveal significant nuanced complexities.

Lythcott also applauds the work being done by Krieger and her colleagues. She thinks that it is important to focus on how mutations themselves can be environmentally created; that black women may suffer
mutations that are not simply biogenetic but rather environmentally
produced specifically through racism and poverty. Lythcott told me of
the new Jean Sindab Afro-American Breast Cancer Research Project at
the Mailman School and the "African-American Breast Cancer Sum-
mit," scheduled for September 2000, organized to address black
women's experience of breast cancer and map a national action plan.
Meanwhile, the long-standing Black Women's Health Project continues

100 to work on health prevention issues for black women and hopes to increase their participation in clinical trials.

The Arthur Ashe Institute for Urban Health has recently devised outreach programs to deal with educating black women about breast cancer. According to Nicole Brown of the Institute, the initiative "Black Pearls" uses existing neighborhood networks established through hair salons to reach black women. At first, ten salon sites were earmarked in East New York and Brownsville, and then eleven more were started in Flatbush and Fort Greene.

## Carcinogenic Capitalism

The average american dumps about four pounds of garbage daily. Trash has become an export. It costs $40 billion a year to get rid of waste, while millions of people go hungry. Landfills and recycling programs are now big business.[36] Corporate america realizes that there are some environmental limits to reckon with, and it has done so within the trajectories of global capital.

Wal-Mart had sales of over $118 billion in 1998, which is larger than the GDP of more than two-thirds of the countries across the globe. Meanwhile children in bangladesh are paid as little as eight cents an hour to sew jeans for Wal-Mart. This too sets the environmental context in which breast cancer as a disease thrives while context and cause are not the same thing.

Corporate america and its ties to global capital structure the artifices of disease in the twenty-first century. The frames of reference that embrace excessive wealth, blame the poor for their lot, seek to limit the public responsibilities of government and corporations alike, and continue to boast of the deregulation and takeover of once public spaces by private corporations define the environments in which the breast cancer establishment now operates.

The breast cancer establishment—which houses the different institutions that do research, study detection, initiate treatment, and provide advocacy—exists alongside and inside the petro/chemical-pharmaceutical/cosmetic complex. The postindustrial medical complex is also

funded through government agencies like the National Institutes of 101
Health and the Environmental Protection Agency. Other times the
funding goes in the reverse direction.[37] This messy rhizomed knot over-
sees and constructs breast cancer discourse.

Some of the very same corporate interests, like Monsanto and
Zeneca, that assault the health of our environments fund cancer research. The cancer establishment is compromised by this relationship
in insidious ways. It often finds itself beholden to chemical and pharmaceutical companies as well as pesticide manufacturers for funding.
Needed research monies build their own compromises. Federal cancer
agencies are linked with the chemical industry and pharmaceutical interests in the makeup of their governing boards and their financial networks.[38] Self-interest conspires and covers over the risks of these
industrial pollutants.

The cancer establishment's institutional base is located in the American Cancer Society, the National Cancer Institute, the Federal Drug
Administration, the Environmental Protection Agency, the Department
of Agriculture, and sectors of the American Medical Association.[39] Together they network to articulate a cohesively authoritative breast cancer
narrative. The cancer establishment favors cure over prevention,
patentable and/or synthetic chemicals over natural and holistic methods. The contours and monies for research follow from this reference
point.

The American Medical Association has strong ties to pharmaceutical companies, and the American Cancer Society owns half of the
patent rights of chemotherapy drugs. There is extraordinary interplay
between the doctors who administer treatments, the scientists who do
the research and set the trials, and the companies that sell the drugs.
The FDA, NCI, and ACS all collaborate on treatments of choice, therapies, and diagnosis.[40]

The Sloan-Kettering Institute for Cancer Research was established
in 1945 with corporate money. The major corporate players offering the
assistance were General Motors, the Rockefellers, and the Morgan
Guaranty Trust. Sloan was president and Kettering was vice-president of
GM.[41] This level of vested interest compromises scientific paradigms

102   and limits the possibility of an interactional biogenetic/environmental science. Breast Cancer Awareness Month (BCAM) reflects this troublesome overlap between the cancer establishment and the postindustrial-medical and petro/chemical-pharmaceutical/cosmetic complexes. Awareness Month was initially sponsored by Imperial Chemical Industries, which was a $14 billion-a-year multinational maker of pesticides, plastics, organochlorines, and pharmaceuticals. In 1993 one of ICI's corporate conglomerates, the Zeneca Group, split off, and took pharmaceuticals, agrichemicals, and Breast Cancer Awareness Month (BCAM) with it.

Troublesome corporate interests are in play here. Burson-Martseller, a powerful multinational public relations firm, worked on behalf of Zeneca Corporation to kill California proposition 65 which sought to register tamoxifen as a carcinogenic substance; worked on behalf of Exxon Corporation after the Valdez oil spill in Alaska; was hired by Union Carbide to represent it after the accident in Bhopal, india; and is the chief PR firm for Monsanto, the chemical/biotech corporation that developed the bovine growth hormone.[42] No wonder that BCAM, funded by Zeneca, has the narrowed focus it does. Zeneca, which retains control over the message of BCAM, publicizes early detection through mammography. In the meantime, mammography has become a million-dollar industry unto itself. And Zeneca makes $300 million a year from sales of the carcinogenic herbicide acetochlor while marketing the world's best-selling cancer therapy drug.[43]

Government regulatory agencies like the FDA interlock with pharmaceutical/drug companies to determine research initiatives and medical trials. There is no federal oversight of consequence of giant polluters like Dow, Monsanto, DuPont. The ACS is the nation's largest and best-known health research charity, and its board is made up of corporate donors.[44] Tobacco companies have clearly been under siege from the cancer wars, but other corporate villains go scot free.

Then-president Clinton agreed to changes in the Clean Air Act that allowed the production of methyl bromide, a poisonous ozone depleting gas used to kill bugs. It is disturbing to know that the major producers of methyl bromide are located in Arkansas and were contributors to Clin-

ton's campaign coffers.[45] Clinton's administration also established a se-  103
ries of corporate tax breaks for pharmaceutical companies that consoli-
dated their trans-nation-state status.

The troublesome complicity does not end with these governmen-
tal/corporate linkages. There is also a corporate-industrial environmental origin to cancer cells themselves. Industrial cancers were first
discussed as such in the early 1900s. Prudential Insurance Company, in
1915, already recognized certain occupations as more carcinogenic than
others.

Wilhelm Hueper directed the National Cancer Institute's Environmental Cancer Section from 1948 to 1964 and focused on environmental carcinogenesis, chemical carcinogenicity, and industrial
carcinogens. He was a critic of "occupational cancer hazards" and the
exposure to industrial chemicals. He believed that lung cancer was a
hazard of the chromium industry. Hueper was censored by the government for his uranium-mining report, and when he retired in 1964 his job
was abolished.[46]

An environmental movement dedicated to protecting the global
habitat began to have significant impact on federal legislation by the
early 1970s. The first Earth Day was celebrated in 1970, as was the sign-
ing of the Environmental Protection and Clean Air Acts. Richard Nixon
declared a war on cancer in 1971. In 1978 Joseph Califano, then secretary of health, education, and welfare, announced that 20–40 percent of
all cancers could be caused by exposure to six industrial pollutants
found in the workplace.[47] Sadly, this was the beginning of the end of
such initiatives as global capital started to amass more political clout.

By the 1980s and the election of Ronald Reagan, there was a significant turnaround for the environmental movement, as well as a new
antigovernment stance that paved the way for global capital's unac-
countability. Reagan orchestrated and oversaw the downsizing and dismantling of federal environmental and occupational health safety
agencies. This assault has left individuals with less of everything: less
protection, less access to health, less ability to better themselves.

This downward spiral for most people across the globe is part and parcel of the accelerated upward spiral of global capital. The less regulation

104    and protection of our environments—be it air, or workplace, or racism —the more egregious the assault on the health of our bodies. As the postindustrial-medical complex becomes more central to the power base of a service economy, it privileges the needs of petro/chemical-pharmaceutical/cosmetic corporate interests that overlap with its own. The overlapping rhizomed knots of power make it harder than ever to resist the profit-driven agenda of global capital.

### Politicized/Cancerous Environments

As a discourse, cancer speaks a naturalized inevitability much like capitalism since the revolutions of 1989. The genetic narrative of cancer nurtures this notion even further. And even when the environment is considered to play a part in the etiology of cancer, it too becomes part of this narration. The environment—and the damage to it—is too complex, too big, for us to be able to turn things around. Cancer narratives depoliticize: if it is our genes we are doomed; if it is our environments we are helpless. Given this, there is not much to be done.

This personal psychic stance nibbles away at our ability to believe in and build political alternatives. However, a few researchers do believe that as much as 60–90 percent of cancers are avoidable in that they are fully a result of exposure to toxic chemicals.[48] I wonder why even I sometimes have trouble believing this. Maybe it is because of Sarah and Giah.

Cancer incidence rose by nearly 25 percent in the u.s. between 1973 and 1991. In this same period the cancer rate of females over sixty-five rose nearly 40 percent, while the incidence in black females of all ages rose more than 30 percent. Given cancer incidence rates, about 40 percent of men and women will contract cancer sometime within their life span.

Exposure to toxic chemicals destroys the respiration of normal cells, depriving them of energy, and damages chromosomes, causing mutations.[49] Studies show that the blood in breast cancer patients contains 35 percent more DDE (a form of metabolized DDT) than that of healthy women.[50] This carcinogen is manmade so it can be unmade. Before carcinogens can be banned they must be seen as detrimental to a normal, healthy way of life. Chemicals like asbestos, benzene, coal tar pitch, vinyl chloride, and iron oxide appear to be unhealthy. There is no safe amount for usage of these chemicals because environmental carcinogens interact with genetic, endocrine, immunological, viral, and physiological factors. What one body can consume with little known harm can kill another.[51] It is hard to know exactly what is going on in any one body because environmental contamination is incremental and continual, much like the process of malignant cell growth.

You are at high cancer risk if you live on the northeast coast, in the Great Lakes area, or near the mouth of the Mississippi River where industrial activity is most intense. High rates of mortality also exist in these regions. In the early 1980s, women residents of Long Island, New York, had breast cancer rates that were 10 to 20 percent higher than the rates in the rest of New York State. In 1994, the New York State Department of Health found a significant correlation between cancer and one's proximity to chemical industrial facilities. High rates of breast cancer on Cape Cod have been connected to contaminated drinking water.[52]

Heredity is rarely the explanation for breast cancer. Yet Sandra Steingraber says that one would think we are sprouting new cancer genes, given the dominant narratives and discourses. The discovery of the BRCA1 and 2 genes tells us too little for a very small number of women. Although initially researchers thought the BRCA1 and 2 genes meant that you had an 85–90 percent chance of developing the disease, just two years later they reformed these estimates to range between 50 and 75 percent. In the first year the women being tested came from families with very high levels of incidence. The sample has widened to include women with lesser levels of familial occurrence. As the sample of women has widened, so has the possibility increased that one can have the gene and not develop breast cancer. So the issue of our environments still remains crucial even in these cases.[53]

Whereas the breast cancer rate is five times higher in the u.s. than in japan, japan's rate is rising more quickly as japan's economy becomes more like the u.s economy. Environmental impact plays a large part here. It explains why japanese women who have moved to the u.s. have

106   the same cancer rates as u.s. women. This is also true of jewish women who immigrate from North Africa (where breast cancer is rare) to israel, a nation with high incidence. Within thirty years after migrating, African-born and israeli-born jews have identical breast cancer rates. If one moves to a country with a lower rate of occurrence, one is subject to the risks attributed to the new home country.[54] This says breast cancer is at least as much about environs as about genes.

If our bodies are part and parcel of our environs, then lifetime exposure to estrogen itself must be contextualized accordingly. Estrogen is produced inside the female body *and* there are chemicals that can act like estrogen that affect the body. These latter xenoestrogens—which are synthetic chemicals that mimic natural estrogens—also blur the contours of female bodies and their environments.

Phthalates, the most abundant plasticized industrial contaminant, has been identified as estrogenic.[55] So I need a science that better recognizes multiple estrogens and an economy that is not based in plastics. And I also want more attention to non-estrogen-triggered breast cancers.

I have rhizomed the body with its surroundings. By seeing and naming the environments that construct breast cancer more complexly and inclusively, we can shape a politics demanding the health of all of our bodies. The breast as a site of "place-consciousness" is my intimate location for this resistance.

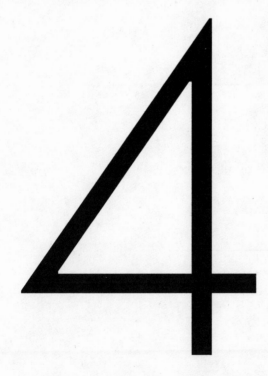

Politicized Environs and
Personal Breasts

# Radicalizing the Pink-Ribboned
# Breast for Us All

S OCIAL, CULTURAL, VISUAL, AND HISTORICAL
contexts continually redefine female bodies. Each definition simultaneously privileges the male body as the standard. This privileging is sym-
bolized by the phallus: the representation of male power via his body.
Women become less than (without a penis), different from; pregnancy
becomes a disability.[1]

Women's breasts symbolize femininity.[2] The breast is in part a masculinist construction of both fact and fiction; physically real and male
fantasy. Most feminisms mean to displace this phallocratic reductionism
of women to their physicality—be it their breasts or their hormones.

Commercial fetishization of breasts and the overstated estrogen narrative contaminate the supposed scientific discourses of breast cancer.
Each woman's breast cancer is unique to her own circumstances and
also shared with other women, while it is problematically universalized
by a masculinist culture that denies the diversity among women.

110     Breast cancer is no one thing. Its meanings circulate in complicated patterns. Culture plays as much a part as nature in its articulation. Advice is marketed with little respect for the complexity and variability of the disease. An oversimplified cause/effect model isolates genes and hormones from their environmental surroundings. Rhizomed relations are falsely bifurcated. This manmade science is overly determined by a biostatic reductionism. Neither genes nor estrogens can be fully understood from this standpoint.

This staticized model of the female body offers women who can afford them mammograms, designer drugs, genetic testing, and tamoxifen. The postindustrial-medical/beauty complex plays a key role in constructing this agenda. The pathways between female bodies, the medical power complex, and the breast cancer establishment are not linear. Nor is the relationship between these power locations and progressive breast cancer activists. There is no singular site of origin but rather a confounding maze.

*Manmade Breast Cancers*

In order to see how breast cancer is manmade, its various environments must be uncovered as part of the setting for science.[3] Masculinist fantasies equate the body with its breasts and ovaries. One sees this in sculpture from prehistoric times. Breasts distinguish the female. They are the outer symbol of femininity. As one explores Pablo Picasso's art one looks for the breasts to find the woman.

The breast as a symbol is disconnected from the ducts and tissue that physically constitute it. The symbolic breast infiltrates the flesh and becomes as cultural as it is biological.

Breast cancer involves gene mutation and out-of-control cell division and proliferation. DNA (deoxyribonucleic acid) transfers genetic information from one generation to the next and forms the building blocks. Inappropriate replication affects millions of diseased cells that have damage to their DNA. Mutated cells, or what are called oncogenes, have to be controlled in order to avoid tumor formation. However, these processes take place within women's bodies, which exist

in multiple environments. And these processes are researched by scientists who occupy particular cultural sites.

Trillions of cells make up the body's system. Old cells are continually replaced, and tumor suppressor genes orchestrate this process. They
signal stop and go to damaged cells. If the suppressor genes are unable
to stop the transmission of damaged DNA to other cells, additional mutations will continue to accumulate.[4] One can inherit a mutation, but it
must be sparked on its journey as an oncogene. The spark or series of
sparks ignites a process that develops over time and expresses different
aspects of environmental input.

Environments play a crucial part in the sequence of cancer mutations.[5] Between 90 and 95 percent of all breast cancers are *not* genetically inherited *and* roughly one-half of women who have inherited the
BRCA1 gene will not develop breast cancer.[6] As well, more than 70 percent of breast cancers are sporadic with no known family history.[7] Environmentally manmade aspects of the disease need much greater
attention.[8]

"Manmade" means that breast cancer is not an inevitable or simply
natural process. Manmade is not the same as male-defined. "Man"
means not natural, but cultural and culture is structured through patriarchal privilege. Female scientists as well as male scientists can be beholden to the linearity and staticity of masculinist science.[9]

"Manmade" also sometimes simply means: inhabited and run by
men. It was not until Bill Young's mother became gravely ill with
metastatic breast cancer that he succeeded in pushing his company,
Genentech, to proceed with trials of the neu protein. The neu protein,
researched by Dennis Slamon, has special growth ferocity as an agent
that the oncogene uses to transform a normal cell to a cancer cell. Slamon had pushed hard for Genentech trials with no success.[10] Young got
the results. This is hardly an objective process fueling research. Thank
goodness for the personal.

"Manmade" also calls attention to the masculinist standards that
deny recognition of the female body. Dr. Susan Love critiques contem-
porary medical approaches for their insensitivity toward women. She vo-
calized what many in the women's health movement were articulating:

112  that the standard breast cancer procedures of "slash, burn, and poison"—mastectomy, radiation, and chemotherapy—were unacceptable to women. She has become an important advocate of lumpectomy and believes in taking extraordinary measures to preserve the breast.[11]

There are biogenetic cells *and* manmade women's bodies, and neither are self-determining if this means they have an autonomous capacity to write their own script. Popularized narratives of breast cancer oversimplify what is *really* known and substitute statistical probabilities for real knowledge. Risk factors are discussed but in highly individualist and nonenvironmentalist form. Detection stands in for prevention.

There is increasing surveillance of women's bodies through new forms of medicalization, like mammography and pap smears.[12] But cancer detection is unevenly available to women. Screening possibilities need to be developed in more varied forms. "Culturally appropriate cues" could help prompt hispanic women to seek out breast cancer screening.[13]

The dominant cultural codes of much breast cancer discourse exclude latino and black women in particular. Most of the outreach and data applies to white middle-class women. The American Cancer Society, in 1988, estimated that approximately 174,000 of all deaths related to malignancy—including breast cancer—might have been prevented by earlier diagnosis and prompt treatment.[14] The lack of outreach and available diagnostic treatment for large numbers of poor women across racial divides has become a part of the etiology of the disease itself.

### EstroGENE Risk and Breast Cancer

Breast cancer is *thought* to be related to high lifetime exposure to estrogen. It is *thought* that estrogen exposure explains approximately 30 percent of breast cancers. Hence, "well-established risk factors" are defined as early menarche, late menopause, family history, late age at first birth. All of these "well-established risk factors" are related to the increase or decrease of estrogen. Even though environmental effects are often recognized as significant in the development of the "multistep process of malignant tumor development," they are not termed risks per

se. When environmental factors are discussed, the lack of scientific evi-   113
dence suggests that they may play a minor role.[15]

Estrogen, as a master narrative of breast cancer, needs much
scrutiny. It smothers important inquiry because there is non-estrogen-receptor breast disease *and* because it parades as a naturalized/hormonal
explanation of what is also an environmental process. There is much to
be unpacked here.

It is noteworthy that even the Program on Breast Cancer and Environmental Risk Factors (BCERF) in New York State, which does such
important work studying and publicizing environmental consequences
of the disease, sometimes inadvertently defers to the estrogen metanarra-
tive. BCERF information materials treat estrogen levels as a known risk
factor, yet do not classify environmental carcinogens as such. Its literature shifts from a language of risk when writing of estrogen, to a standard
of noncausality when discussing environment. This shift reflects two
quite different standards of evaluation.

BCERF's fact-finding has been crucial in establishing the long-term
effects of harmful pesticides that remain active and stored in soil for
years after their application and use even if they are not recognized as
part of the immediate danger.[16] It is also important to note, however,
that most breast cancer is not attributable to the large array of established risk factors to begin with. Only 21 percent of premenopausal and
29 percent of postmenopausal breast cancers are related to one or more
risk factors.[17]

Some environmental scientists attempt to complicate the estrogen
narrative. Environmental effects—both inside and outside the body—
are necessary in order to fully appreciate estrogen levels in the first
place. Endogenous estrogens are just part of the story. So replace the
biostatic view of estrogen and proceed with interactional research studies that deal with the flows between different environmental pollutants.
Break open the divide between genes and environment and recognize
the multistep and long-term interactional process of malignant cells.
Then risk becomes a rhizomed affair and harm is understood in preventive ways that move beyond the staticized view of estrogen.[18] Then the
environment is no longer posed against the hormone estrogen.

*Risking Environmental Aging*

Breast cancer risk is multifactorial, multimechanistic, and multi-stage. Yet I. Craig Henderson says that age might be the single most important factor.[19] Age, in this instance, bespeaks multiple factors—the longer we breathe foul air, the longer we live with environmental racism, the longer we are exposed to endogenous and exogenous hormones, the less the body can cope and repair itself.

Only 6 percent of breast cancers in the u.s. are in women under age forty.[20] Most breast cancer—almost 80 percent— is in women over fifty; but breast cancer is the leading cause of death of women between forty and forty-four years old.[21] One's risk of developing breast cancer is most often expressed after the age of seventy-five.[22] One-quarter of the women who die of breast cancer are over sixty-five years of age.[23] More than 75 percent of breast cancers diagnosed in the u.s. each year are in women over fifty years of age. It is important to know that a majority of breast cancers occur in women over fifty because this means that for most women it takes a good portion of their lifetime to succumb to malignancy. Since this is the case for most women, it is important to develop the etiology of breast cancer from a life-course perspective—in part carefully studying the significance of adolescent hormonal changes—with an environmental standpoint.

The shorthand statistical statement—that one out of every eight women will get breast cancer—distorts more than clarifies individual risk. Risk for women by age twenty-five is one in 19,608; by age thirty-five it is one in 622; by age forty-five one in 93; by age seventy-five one in 11. One must live to be eighty-five to reach the 1 in 8 risk level.[24]

Women *become* more susceptible as they age. Breast cancer, then, has a history that develops over time through a series of life events. In the u.s., breast cancer incidence from 1970 to 1990 increased almost 40 percent for women sixty-five or older, but increased less than 5 percent for women younger than fifty.[25]

It is now hypothesized that breast cancer can be in process from as little as three years to as much as thirty-five years before malignancy is detectable.[26] This recognition of a process developing over time should spark new inquiry about long-term prevention.

I remember when I first learned how long malignant growth may take. I tried to imagine how old I might have been when my cancer began. It felt so strange to realize that my breast cancer was already in progress while I was pregnant and breastfeeding my daughter. I keep wondering what this might mean for her. Charles, my oncologist, says this in itself means little, but we both know he does not really know.

Given this long-term process, it is almost already too late to advise women to have mammograms at age forty if one is *really* committed to prevention. A proactive long-term public health stance is needed. Breast cancer initiatives must address the health of the multiple environments of the female body while especially targeting adolescent girls. Demand healthy breasts by transforming the environments we inhabit.

There is evidence that suggests that developing breast tissue is particularly vulnerable to environmental toxins, some of which operate as xenoestrogens. During this time of breast development it may be particularly important to safeguard young women from carcinogenic exposure. So girls should be encouraged to take a proactive posture toward their bodies through healthful eating and exercise. This is no easy task when adolescent girls are so deeply burdened by their own sense of vulnerability, in part defined by the larger masculinist and racist culture they occupy. A balance must be struck between girls' fear of breast cancer and their taking action to prevent it; between protecting their bodies and enhancing them. Girls also need more than a personal politics in this instance, because there is no individual solution to the breast cancer problem.

Breast Cancer Awareness Month advertises early detection by mammography as the best prevention. Detection finds, but does not prevent, disease.[27] Early-stage detection most often increases your chances of survival, and this is no small thing. But mammography should not be confused with what it is not. Besides, the mammogram message does not apply to adolescent girls or young women with their dense breast tissue.

My family's story increases my skepticism of mammography because mammograms do not always do what they are supposed to do. My sister Sarah discovered the lump in her breast herself; it never showed on

116 X-ray. Neither did either of my sister Giah's breast tumors. When I first met with my surgeon, he requested that I have a mammogram so he could better know the dimensions of the tumor. It was not depicted in the film. Mammography fails to detect breast cancer in approximately 20 percent of women over fifty and in 40 percent of younger women.

For sure, mammograms sometimes make sense and save lives. But they are not good enough as a screening device for women under forty, and are not foolproof for older women either. And they are not a sensible option for young women like my daughter, because it is not at all clear what the long-term effects of repetitive mammography are. There needs to be more discovery and testing of alternatives like thermography, which measures infrared-sensitive material through heat, or video machines that illuminate the breast by using high-intensity light, or ultrasound to search for tissue abnormalities, or protection of the breast with melatonin before X-ray.[28] And there must be access for all women to whatever forms of detection there are. Just now, in Texas, which has the highest percentage of women without health insurance of any state, four in ten women over fifty have not had a mammogram in the last two years.

Breast cancer rates have increased at 1 percent a year since the 1940s.[29] More women have died of breast cancer in the past two decades than all Americans killed in World War I, World War II, the Korean War, and the Vietnam War combined. There are 182,000 new cases diagnosed each year.[30] Detection, by itself, and with no guarantee of access, is simply not a coherent strategy.

## Risking Racism

Organochlorines—pollutants which are fat soluble—accumulate and persist in human tissue. Nancy Krieger and her colleagues have found that higher serum levels of organochlorines exist for black women.[31] In 1984 probabilities for developing breast cancer by the age of seventy-five varied along racial lines. For whites it was a 1 in 12, for blacks 1 in 14, for japanese americans 1 in 19. Yet black women die more often than white women from breast cancer.[32]

According to Krieger a review of the literature indicates that breast cancer has risen the most rapidly among young women who are black and/or poor. There was a slightly earlier age of menarche for black women but with small effect. Teenage pregnancy has been up for whites and down for blacks since 1970. So although there is a rise of breast cancer among young black women, there is low attributable risk from most known risk factors.[33] Do hormones play a part here?

Krieger is not intimidated by questions she cannot answer. She wonders what the extent of exposure is to exogenous carcinogens. She wonders about the kind of susceptibility breast tissue has to these exposures. Can infants and children drinking milk and eating foods with fat-soluble carcinogens accumulate these substances in their breast tissue as a start toward malignant changes of breast cells? Does susceptibility heighten around puberty owing to breast tissue growth? Do additional exposures, including endogenous reproductive hormones, continue the process toward malignancy?

It may be that there are specific carcinogenic exposures along with unique reproductive histories that instigate breast cancer in tandem with each other. In this scenario, exposure and one's body's susceptibility create a complex nexus. Krieger even wonders whether exogenous nonhormonal exposures—rather than endogenous hormones—play the primary role in breast cancer risk. In part this would explain why in migration studies—from poland, japan, central america to the u.s.—breast cancer risk is highest among those who migrated *prior* to adulthood.[34]

Krieger also notes the persistent trend that for women under the age of forty the incidence of breast cancer is higher for blacks than for whites. She hypothesizes that this incidence level can be explained by a shifting combination of exposure and susceptibility. Age-specific breast cancer represents a set of complex class relations that are shaped by race. Krieger also initially wondered whether abortion rates increase susceptibility to exogenous carcinogenic exposures. Then abortion patterns *and* community and home-based carcinogenic exposures would explain a higher incidence of breast cancer among young working-class women.[35] This initial hypothesis was not borne out, but Krieger continues to study the intersections of age, race, and class.

*Genes and Environmental Genetics*

Given how rare hereditary breast cancer is, it is amazing how many people believe the genetics narrative. Much of the power of this narrative derives from the individualist biostatic viewing of the body. From this stance, people are one and the same with their genes.

It is true that one's statistical chances of getting breast cancer rise to an 80 percent risk if one's mother has had it; and increase even further, to a 130 percent risk, if a sister has.[36] But, once again, this is not just simply about genes.

Familial breast cancer may be both inherited *and* acquired. When there is a genetic disposition to develop breast cancer, environment continually plays a part. Sisters are more likely to share similar environments for a longer period of time and through their adolescent years. Maybe this explains the higher risk of having a sister with breast cancer than a mother.

This ecogenetics—a mix of genetic potential and possibility that is defined by the particular context—recognizes the importance of individual bodies *and* their need for safety in the air, food, and water they depend on.[37] Genetic susceptibility rather than genetic determination demands safe environments.

Breast cancer cells are made. The process of cell damage leading to malignancy is not a completely in-house affair. If it was, then every woman with a BRCA gene would get breast cancer.

So, for most women, breast cancer is more acquired than inherited. Many studies find that levels of PCBs and DDT are 50 to 60 percent higher in the breast tissue of women with breast cancer than in women without.[38] Nassau and Suffolk Counties in New York State have higher levels of breast cancer, probably owing to the proximity of toxic dumpsites, polluted water, and old asbestos water pipes.

Environmental scientists adopt this estrogen visor when they discuss some pollutants as estrogen mimics. These pesticides are likened to estrogen because molecularly they look like estrogen to the body, including all its estrogen-positive cancer cells.

These synthetic exogenous estrogens damage the balance between 119 one's natural endogenous estrogen and cell replication. They are man-made hormonelike pollutants that act like human hormones and fool the body as such. The bovine growth hormone found in milk, rbST, is thought to act in such a fashion.

There is also research that begins to show that plant or phytoestrogens can interfere in the processes of harmful xenoestrogens. Phytoestrogens can work against malignant growth by occupying the receptor sites of breast, ovary, and other tissue so the "real" estrogen or the estrogen mimics will not be able to take up residence. Phytoestrogens can also interfere with enzymes that are necessary for cancer growth. Soy, tofu, whole grains, and fiber are thought to function in this fashion.

I still wonder about Sarah and Giah and the pill. And whether Julia will be spared breast cancer because she does not have the BRCA1 gene; or not. I wonder when I am tested for the BRCA gene what it will mean for my daughter.

## The So-Called Science of Estrogen

Constructs of femininity imagine the female body as one and the same with its breasts and its ovaries. Estrogen, produced largely by the ovaries, becomes culturally embroiled in this biogenetic construction of breast cancer. Estrogen, as a female hormone, as what makes women different from men, is singled out for particular scrutiny. Masculinist culture seeps into the scientific environment here through a series of unexamined sites.

It is thought that estrogen *may* play a role in creating breast cancer by stimulating breast cell division. Even literature that assumes that estrogen is a major culprit uses the qualifying phrase: "maybe" estrogen feeds breast cancer cells. But the "maybe" gets forgotten, and breast cancer is spoken of as estrogen dependent.

The linkage between one's menstrual cycle and the probability of developing breast cancer is taken as well established. Usually by the age of ten, ovaries begin making estrogen.[39] It is thought by some

120   researchers that each year menarche is delayed, the subsequent risk of
breast cancer is decreased by 20 percent.[40] The average age of menstrua-
tion in china is seventeen; menopause is forty-eight. In india young
women usually menstruate around fourteen years of age.[41] But by what
mechanisms has estrogen become the dominant focus for this research
when such variety exists?

It is often said that lesbians are at higher risk for breast cancer because they do not bear children. Of course this assumes that lesbians
have not had children, which is very often not the case. So is the assumption of lesbian high risk simply, an assumption, or is there evidence to the contrary? As well, if lesbians are found to have higher
cancer rates, is it not possible that one's economic status is also in play
here? Maybe some lesbians suffer the absence of male wages like poor
women more generally.[42]

What part does the cultural environment of science play in establishing hormonal, and therefore reproductive, factors as the clearest risk
for breast cancer? Breast cancer data distinguish between pre- and postmenopausal women, but menopause in and of itself is a long-term
process of hormonal changes rather than a singular event. So what does
pre- and postmenopausal mean in this instance? To begin with, there is
no one kind of menopause. Patricia Kaufert argues that considerable
heterogeneity exists among women within the category menopausal.[43]

There most probably is always some environmental and interactional impact on endogenous estrogen. Maybe this is *in part* why
menopause—as the eventual cessation of estrogen—is so varied in its expressions. Margaret Lock says that menopause is a product of what she
terms "local knowledge."[44] In the u.s., instead of seeing variety in mid-
dle-aged women, we see estrogen levels, hot flashes, and future heart attacks. Women in japan experience menopause, which is most closely
approximated in the term "konenki," somewhat differently. It is viewed
more as a change of life, but not a distressing one. Japanese women will
sometimes speak of "hot feelings" but not often. Only 10 percent in one
study complained of hot flashes in the way they are depicted by many
u.s. women. Only 4 percent mentioned night sweats.[45]

Breast cancer, also, expresses itself differently across countries and across environments of class and race. This should be enough to query a notion of estrogen as a biostatic entity shared by all females alike. Obviously, female bodies vary among themselves: no two are identical, nor do they share exact amounts of estrogen because this varies according to where and how they live. And where and how they live affects breast cancer incidence.

Whereas one woman in one thousand is diagnosed with breast cancer in the u.s., this is true for one woman in ten thousand in algeria.[46] Breast cancer is the number-one cause of death in israel, with jewish women at greatest risk, while ashkenazi and russian immigrants are at greater risk than their sephardi and ethiopian sisters.[47]

I query the naturalized and static viewing of estrogen. I reject its homogeneous construction because it varies in amount, and origin, and constancy. These variations shift according to diet, which is also culturally, racially, and economically constructed. Estrogen needs to be studied, but in its contextual form, taking account of its variability, changeability, and unknowability.

Given all the focus on estrogen, I should remind you that only "one to two-thirds of all breast tumors have estrogen receptors and depend on estrogen for growth."[48] This means that anywhere from one to two-thirds of breast tumors are not thought to be estrogen dependent. One to two-thirds means that a minority of breast cancers might be estrogen fed. Also, the designation one to two-thirds does not sound very exact or scientific to me.

In 1973, at the time my sister Sarah was diagnosed, there was no test in place to decipher one's receptor status. Her doctors, nevertheless, working from the estrogen model, suggested a prophylactic hysterectomy. Desperate for anything that might save her life, she agreed. She died five years later. Neither Giah's nor my breast cancer was estrogen receptor sensitive.

I do not know if I would have become skeptical of the dominance of the estrogen model if my family's story were different. Or whether I would have been as critical of the false clarity that is assumed by this stance. Nonetheless, I wonder what the full effects of this viewing are, and how it limits the exploration of the varieties of breast cancer.

122    Maybe most disturbing about this estrogen story line is that it cata-
pults tamoxifen to the center of breast cancer treatment and so-called
prevention.

### The Estrogen-Tamoxifen Connection

Tamoxifen was developed by the London-based Imperial Chemical Industries. The World Health Organization in 1996 designated tamoxifen a human carcinogen.[49] According to Dr. Janette Sherman it
shares a similar biochemical action to DDT and methoxychlor and di-
ethylstilbestiol, better known as DES. She believes that tamoxifen sub-
stitutes one disease for several others in healthy women while possibly
prolonging survival and decreasing recurrence in women with breast
cancer.[50] Yet tamoxifen is marketed to these two different groups:
healthy women at high risk in the hopes of prevention *and* women with
breast cancer.

In April 1998 the National Cancer Institute announced that its trials
of tamoxifen had shown it to be a preventive for breast cancer decreasing the risk by 45 percent for those involved in the clinical study.[51] In
September 1998 the Food and Drug Administration voted unanimously
to recommend approval of the drug tamoxifen to "reduce women's risk"
of developing breast cancer. The drug would be marketed for women
only at "high risk" but was still seen as a milestone in the effort to *prevent* cancer.[52]

The promise of tamoxifen is based on the notion that it reduces estrogen levels, that it lessens the effect of estrogen, that it is an estrogen
blocker and starves estrogen-fed/fueled breast cancer, that it inhibits estrogen and therefore the growth of cancer cells.[53] In sum, the less estrogen, the less breast cancer. Tamoxifen acts as an antiestrogen by binding
to estrogen receptors located in cancerous cells, preventing the trigger-
ing of the cells.

Meanwhile, estrogen replacement therapy (ERT) for menopausal
women is also said to be scientifically safe and not to create a greater risk
of breast cancer. ERT is heralded as a plus for menopausal women, eas-
ing hot flashes and mood swings and protecting the heart. However, in

April 2000, a federal study of hormone replacement therapy found that  123
ERT, instead of protecting the heart, puts women at slightly higher risk
of heart attacks and strokes.[54]

The National Cancer Institute trial of tamoxifen included 13,388
women. Of these women, 85 who were taking tamoxifen developed
breast cancer, compared with 154 who were not. Hence the finding of a
45 percent reduction. Thirty-three women taking tamoxifen developed
cancer of the uterine lining, whereas 14 women taking the placebo did.
Seventeen women on tamoxifen developed blood clots in their lungs,
while 6 on the placebo did. Meanwhile, several british and italian tamoxifen studies have found no reduction in breast cancer risk.[55]

It remains a key question which women are at high enough risk—
however risk is defined here—to benefit from tamoxifen, while tens of
millions of women could be said to be worthwhile candidates. When
does one risk the health of a healthy woman by exposing her to a carcinogenic as a preventive method? Frances Visco, president of the National Breast Cancer Coalition (NBCC), responds to the FDA's ruling
by saying that she is cautiously optimistic about tamoxifen as a preventive treatment for high-risk women.[56]

The National Women's Health Network presents an aggressive indictment of tamoxifen and its drug trials. Their report, "Tamoxifen for
Prevention," queries the real essence of the findings. The report states
that although 2.3 percent of the women taking the placebo developed
breast cancer, while 1.27 percent on tamoxifen did, this is not a big
enough difference to justify the use of a carcinogenic drug on healthy
women. This 1 percent difference is translated into a 45 percent reduction in risk. Besides this, there is no proof that tamoxifen prevents death.
In the trial five women died who were taking tamoxifen (three from
cancer, two from pulmonary embolisms) and five women died (from
cancer) taking the placebo.[57]

Tamoxifen creates a higher risk for uterine cancer and blood clots. It
can cause ocular toxicity, leading to retinal impairment. The advantages
are assumed to be greatest for women over fifty, but these women are
also at greater risk for these side effects.

Little is understood about how tamoxifen works. The trials give

124 statistical evidence that reflect probabilities, not scientific understanding. Tamoxifen is *thought* to act by "competing with estrogen for estrogen receptors in the nuclei of the cells of *some* breast cancers." It is said to *maybe* inhibit the metabolism of breast cancer cells.[58] But all we have here is a statement that tamoxifen is thought to work on some cancers. We do not know which cancers, nor do we definitively know much else.

What about the drug trial itself? None of the data warrant a wholesale endorsement for women across racial and class lines, given the racial and class homogeneity of the sampling. And high risk is a problematic category. It obviously will be defined more widely than the rough 5 percent of women thought to have the BRCA1 and 2 genes.

Within one year's time new information from the National Cancer Institute (NCI) has shown that tamoxifen is not the panacea promised. Much of what the Women's Health Network initially cautioned has been verified by the NCI itself. A recent publication by the NCI says that almost all women over the age of sixty are more likely to be harmed than helped by using tamoxifen prophylactically. Younger women are at lesser risk of complication, but still face serious problems. The outcomes for african-american women sixty and older are also negative.[59] And according to the Women's Health Network, high-risk white women in their forties are more likely to experience an overall benefit than african-american women in this age group.[60]

Tamoxifen is designed to be taken daily for a five-year regime. It costs between $80 and $100 a month. Sales already totaled $320 million in 1997, and this was before the FDA approved it as a preventive drug.[61] The postindustrial-medical complex has woven a complex directorate of implicit deceit and misrepresentation of the estrogen-breast cancer-tamoxifen connection. Environmental biogenetics has been crowded out by a medical politics deeply embedded in pharmaceutical and chemical corporations hell-bent on selling an estrogen blocker that itself may be carcinogenic.

Breast cancer is big business. Many of the same corporations that contaminate our bodily environments sell the drugs that are supposed to prevent malignancy. Zeneca manufactures pesticides at the one end and

markets tamoxifen at the other. The postindustrial-medical/beauty com-    125
plex researches and markets breast cancer at the same time. This just
might be a deadly combination: moneymaking and women's health.

My critique of tamoxifen is focused on its claims as a "prevention"
for healthy women who are at high risk. I have much less to say about its
use as a treatment for women with breast cancer because so many of the
treatments to date are possibly carcinogenic and/or problematic for our
overall health. When I took adryamycin I knew beforehand that it could
damage my heart. To this day I cannot know what the long-term impact
has been or will be on my overall health. These unknowns are part of
any breast cancer drug treatment, drugs including but not particular to
tamoxifen.

## Local U.S. Breast Cancer Activism

The many types of feminism are as varied as women's bodies are.
Breast cancer activism also reflects an incredible pluralism. Some breast
cancer activists identify as feminist, others do not. Some came to their
activism through their experience of breast cancer, others were political
beforehand. And some activists are simply committed to women's health
as a politics unto itself.

Feminists of many different origins work at redefining women's bodies' meanings. Women's liberation has sometimes meant freeing woman
*from* her body; other times it has meant freeing women *to* explore and
name their bodies. There are some forms of cultural and radical feminism that have celebrated the female body in its biostatic naturalist
form. Feminist struggles for women's equality often sidestep the body
and focus more on economic and legal equity. No surprise that there are
as many different kinds of feminisms as there are multiple representa-
tions and interpretations of the female body.

Breast cancer activism is inflected with these plural forms of feminism.[62] Much breast cancer advocacy work assumes a liberal individualist approach that women know their bodies best and should partake in
defining their treatments and care. This stance focuses on the individual

126  and her need for information, support, and advocacy. Susan Love's approach is oriented by these concerns. She is very critical of the insensitivity of masculinist medicine and relies on women to help choose their own care. She prefers breast conservation—lumpectomy—because it is as effective as mastectomy and also because she thinks this will make breast cancer less frightening to women. Her approach is both radically critical of patriarchal privilege and radically uncritical of the breast.

Because breast cancer—as a science, as a disease, as a set of protocols—is so imbricated in the cultural and corporatist relations of power, it cannot be cleansed of all its masculinist or commercialized markings. Lumpectomy, as a medical procedure, reflects the importance of women's body parts to themselves and also is deeply wedded to societal preoccupation with the breast. Breast cancer activism absorbs these unclear boundaries of body and culture in its various political strategies.

The breast cancer movement, if one can assume a cohesive coalition of health activists committed to prevention, detection, research, treatment, and advocacy, developed in part from the women's health movement of the 1970s. As a movement it broke the silence surrounding breast cancer and made it noisily visible. There are hundreds of local groups and task forces established around the country dedicated to distributing information, demanding access to mammograms and treatment, and providing support to women living with breast cancer. One of the earliest expressions of this activism was the demand of Long Island women for epidemiological studies of their neighborhoods, given the high rates of incidence there.

There are national groups like the NBCC who give high public visibility to the disease. There are activist groups like the Women's Community Cancer Project in Cambridge, Massachusetts, and the Breast Cancer Fund in San Francisco who radically push for more inclusive understanding and research. Breast cancer activism has matured into a blend of authorized institutionalized activities—focusing on legislation and research funding—and insurgent critiques of the disease itself. Parts of this activist network work in a cautious partnership with the postindustrial-medical complex, while other parts exist in more skeptical relation to it.

Breast cancer activism is committed to empowering women in their
own lives. The well-known early feminist health collective *Our Bod-*
*ies/Ourselves* demanded women's control over their biological destiny;
women speaking for themselves about their own bodies.[63] The consciousness-raising focus of the early women's movement—to share experiences collectively in order to change them—helped to envision the
early breast cancer hot-line networks and support groups. These self-
help groups nurtured women through their fears, their pain, and sometimes their deaths. Women found comfort from knowing there were
others like them, that they were not just alone.[64]

Breast cancer advocacy also had early ties to the AIDS movement.
The pink ribbon, derivative of the red AIDS ribbon, initially sought to
publicize breast cancer by breaking the silence about it. Breast cancer
activism has taken many of its cues from the AIDS movement especially
in terms of demanding more government funding for research.

I wear the pink ribbon pin to make the disease visible in a collective
sense. I wear the pin to connect my individual self to the larger collectiv-
ity of women living with breast cancer. I like the fact that wearing the
pin does not only mean that I, personally, have breast cancer. My cancer
is not just about my own body but involves women as a group more
broadly. This collective identity that I wear publicly is more than simply
personal.

It also troubles me that I purchase the pink pins from Avon cosmetics. I, like many feminists, would have preferred purple pins, to speak
the history of feminism more prominently. But Estee Lauder, the origi-
nator of this campaign, did not ask, so pink it was. Avon's beauty products commercialize women's bodies. Avon sells breast cancer products
bearing the pink ribbon—from pens, to mugs, to key chains—and com-
mercializes bodies at the same time. Although the monies go to research, the research nexus is also embedded in this masculinist and
corporate beauty complex. Avon markets the very notion of femininity
that gets in the way of innovative science. Once again, there is no simple inside and outside in this instance.

Breast cancer activism, reaching full stride in the mid-1980s, was impacted by the privatization and conservatism of the Reagan-Bush decade.

128   With organized feminism under attack, much activism took on the form of an identity politics that sidelined the structural relations of corporatist power. Self-help often wins out as a strategy because insurgent and radical coalitions are hard to develop given the growing power of the cancer establishment and its sometimes complicit relations with the postindustrial-medical complex *and* pharmaceutical/chemical corporations.

Activism often targets single issues, and task forces prioritize their focus: on the environment, on funding for research, on new drug trials, on outreach, on guaranteed health care. The disparate and singular venues reflect the difficulties of developing multiple and radical political agendas today.[65] Breast cancer activism has unfolded in anarchic, individualist, and collective forms. It has developed inside and outside the cancer establishment; and inside and outside the postindustrial beauty complex.[66]

Rose Kushner, who wrote of her mastectomy in *Why Me?* was a member of the National Institutes of Health and a founder of the Breast Cancer Advisory Center. She worked as an advocate for change with the National Cancer Institute and the National Cancer Advisory Board, established by Jimmy Carter in 1980.[67] Representative Mary Rose Oakar was a leader in Congress, establishing money for further research as part of the Public Health Service Act.

Happy Rockefeller, Betty Ford, and Nancy Reagan shared their breast cancers early on with the american public. From a very different cultural location, black feminist Audre Lorde sought to make black women's breast cancer visible. As early as the nineteen fifties, Reach to Recovery was formed to assist women in dealing with their mastectomies. Today breast cancer activists advocate on behalf of women, to find a "cure."

The Race for the Cure, sponsored by Avon, started in 1990. It is now a yearly runners' event held across the country where women with breast cancer, their friends and loved ones, raise awareness and money for research.

The NBCC articulates a legislative agenda that hopes will lead to the eradication of breast cancer. It assumes an "industry partnership" in

its attempt at advocating new funding for research. It has successfully
increased research monies from $90 million in 1990 to $600 million in
2000 under the tutelage of Fran Visco. NBCC also participates in education, legislative initiatives, and policy formation.[68]

The Women's Community Cancer Project, founded in 1989, is radically committed to women's health activism. It openly indicts the corpo-
rate/monied vested interests in breast cancer disease. The Project states
clearly in its literature that Breast Cancer Awareness Month should be
more rightly called National Cancer Industry Awareness Month.[69]

The Breast Cancer Fund's agenda, according to its director, Andrea
Martin, insists on pushing the edge and questioning the status quo of
breast cancer. The Fund recognizes breast cancer as a wedge to the
larger issue of environmental health, insists on more environmental research, pushes for alternatives to mammography, and seeks more reli-
able technologies and the replacement of toxic treatments.[70]

The breast cancer movement is unified in its focus on the disease. It
is disparate in its conception and naming of it. At the center sits the pink
ribbon reminding women to be physically fit, nutritionally healthy, and
savvy about detection.[71] The issues of corporate malfeasance and environmental racism remain at the margins of the more publicized repre-
sentations. So the breast cancer movement needs to enhance a
rhizomatic structure to assist the particular and specific agendas of the
different activist groups while also publicizing the need for a more multiple and opened viewing of the breast's health. This must bring the
complexity of breast disease—with its racial and class aspects—to the
center of the agenda.

Activist groups need to continue focusing on their particular and
differing agendas, but they also need to support coalition work that
moves beyond their specific commitments. Environmental justice
groups need to name breast health as key to their platforms, and breast
cancer activists must herald safer and juster environments. The issues
and tissues of the breast must be connected to the equality of access to
health care. Individual empowerment must be integrated with structural
change.

130    I am back again to the intimate connection of personal and political life. But the personal is never enough, because taken alone, it is too private and singular. Radicalize the pink ribbon by demanding a more specified place-consciousness for us all. I know Sarah, and Giah, and Julia agree.

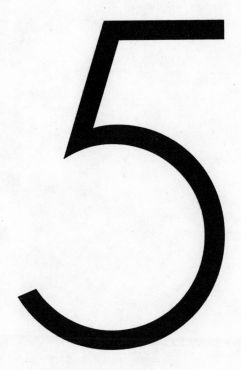

# 5

The Personal Is
Incompletely Political

# Returning to Feminism through the Locale of the Breast

I MAY NEED TO EXPLAIN THIS NEXT TWIST. SO FAR I have looked at the breast through its overlapping—cultural, economic, masculinist, scientific, and racial—environments to see its complexity and changeability. Now I focus more specifically on a few events that shape the political environs and its discourses. So I have shifted from breast cancer in its environs to the political discourses shaping the way we see, or do not want to see, or cannot see this disease. So antigovernment rhetoric, and the Clinton sex scandals, and the u.s. women's soccer team become part of my environmental narrative.

None of this is easily self-evident, so I will tell you a bit of my argument before it unfolds. Given the narrowed sense of governmental responsibility of the Reagan-Bush-Clinton administrations for the past

134  quarter-century, the public sphere has shrunk while the private corporate sector has grown. This process of the shrinking public demands that individuals take more and more responsibility for themselves; and expects less of government. With little sense of the public good, there is little sense of the public health.

This neoliberalism manipulates the demarcations between public and private, and personal and political, for its own purposes of financial gain. Neoliberalism has shrunk the notion of "public," shifted the focus from the political to the personal, and articulated a divide between the two. This disconnect sets a context for bifurcating the complex relations between sex and gender; race and gender and class; nature and culture; breast cancer and its long-term rhizomed context. If the political and public is *not* viewed as personal, then this separation can be used to undermine the connection between things like the body and its effects. It then becomes quite difficult to see the overlap between one's body and its environments.

In this neoliberal view, race is treated more as a biogenetic given than as a culturally defined socioeconomic reality. But if one is to assert that black women's breast cancer is not simply about a biogenetics of race, that race itself is a multifactored multidimensional determinant, then one needs to chart the constructions of whiteness. I make a quick accounting of some very recent formulations of this process with Lizzie Dole and Hillary Rodham.

Because breast cancer is always both personal and political, I look to the particular moment of the Clinton sex scandals to see a rewriting of this feminist claim. The sex scandals were *public*ized across the globe. U.S. politics pollinates outside u.s. borders because it is power-filled by its transnational corporate nexus. So although this is a very local u.s. story, it is also with global effects.

The most localized site is the body. Yet the body is never just a local site because it exists in layers made outside itself. So the body is local and global simultaneously. My local viewing of the health of the breast exists within the locale of u.s. neoliberalism. And this local site also travels and locates elsewhere. Feminisms across the globe suffer for these particular conservative moments.

*Revisiting Feminism and the Breast*

What do I mean when I say I wish to return to feminism at the millennium through the breast? A female breast is a fleshy body part *and* a location of resistance. Breasts can be made into anything we choose, and this is also *not so.*

I write of breasts while women suffer the cultural overidentification with their bodies. My focus on a colored rainbow of bodies celebrates the overwhelming importance of sexual pleasure and bodily health while also rejecting the equation of femaleness with our bodies.

I came to feminism when I was twenty-one years old with all my body parts. At that time I spoke of women with no particular bodily emphasis. But my writing now is *not* from a sense of lacking body parts. Nor do I see the breast as simply a passive site for corporate agendas, pollution, and disease. Rather the breast can also be an empowering place from which to recognize the vulnerability of the human body and demand protection and resources for its health.

Breasts are a reminder of our physicality, of our vulnerability, *and* our potentiality for developing a more complete environmentalist understanding of our bodies. Breast cancer speaks danger while a breast *can* also resonate nurturance, sexuality, and resistance. The breast as body part *and* as a racialized masculinist construction means that it entertains a tense and ambivalent relationship to feminism itself. It therefore is a risky but passionate place to build this consciousness for resistance.

This tension allows feminism the opportunity to rethink the complex relations of the body and its power-filled meanings. Because the female breast absorbs environments and also becomes an environment for transmitting breast milk on the one hand, and masculinist objectification on the other, the breast exists neither simply inside nor simply outside its perceived contours. Nor is it just a personal or a political location. Breasts as part of bodies that are part of racialized genders that are in turn part of the larger political cultures they inhabit disallow clear demarcations between the personal and political, body and culture, sex and gender, color and race.

136     One sees this deep imprint of breast culture maybe most clearly with people who reject the clarity of heterosexist categories of identity. For female to male transsexuals, mastectomy is experienced as freedom. A lesbian friend who nurses her baby says she is constantly misread as straight because she is breast-feeding. Lesbian political demonstrations are sometimes militantly topless, in defiance of cultural mores and the police. Same breasts, many meanings.

If political context always matters for deciphering the meanings of gender, then present-day breast cancer rhetoric that focuses on women as victims must be met skeptically. Feminisms must take the breast and focus attention on the deteriorating political and economic environments of global capitalism for women of all colors, in all locales.

### Revisiting the Personal as Political

As I write from my body toward feminism, and from feminism toward *the* body, I stumble on the tensions between the body's personal and political meanings: between sex and gender, genes and environs, sexualities and heterosexism, color and race.

As I move toward feminism I take my body with me. The dynamism of feminism emanates from the intensity of this connection because the body is as potentially political as it is biogenetic. This is why the political character of the body, as Michel Foucault says, is the first thing that power conceals.[1] It is probably why shorthand phrases like "the personal is political," "the politics of sex," and "sexual politics" have such resilience.

Feminism denies the fantasy that sex, meaning bodies and their sexuality, *and* politics are separate and by doing so rejects the neat divide between private and public life.[2] This understanding also reframes the relations between family and nation and between nation and globe.

But "the personal as political" swallows too much in its phrasing because the personal stands for a variety of meanings. "Personal" can simply mean the individual private self. This self also refers to female biology and its reproductive capacity, its sexual desire and identification, and its bodily health. And these private selves are also publicly webbed.

Each of these meanings is already constructed through the lenses of racialized gender: the cultural interpretations enforcing standards of racialized femininity in its differentiated class meanings.

A public politics of gender infiltrates the privacy of sex and sexuality. So sex is never simply private or personal and yet it is the most private experience we can know. Our bodies parade publicly and yet we live in them utterly singularly. Sex appears to be everywhere and is supposedly open and free, yet most people reveal little of their sex lives to others. Foucault is at his best explaining how constant talk of sex controls us more than it frees us. A key aspect of the Lewinsky scandal supposedly was that it was *not* about sex. Sex is spoken everywhere, yet regulated and disciplined in all the noise.

Sexgate—the lies of Bill Clinton about his affair with Monica Lewinsky—confusingly unraveled the discourse of personal privacy. Bill said that what he did was private and was no one's business but his family's. Monica, the intern Clinton had the affair with, said she felt totally exposed; she was left with no privacy. She felt humiliated. What she had done was meant to be private. No one was to know, not her parents or the public. The exposure left her with nowhere to hide as the public watched. She felt "naked to the whole world." Once Bill finally confessed as president, Monica said she saw only a "selfish man who lies all the time." There was no privacy left, and he finally became in her mind a "politician all the time."[3]

In the postsexgate era, it is no easy task to sort out the relations between personal sex and public politics because they are not equatable or reducible to each other. Sexgate undermined the feminist recognition that there is a politics to sex; that sex in imbricated in and through relations of power. Bill's private acts were deemed unimpeachable, which they probably were. However, this ruling was used to justify a renewed viewing of public and private life as separate and apart. *And* very old ways of speaking about women, sex, and their bodies were validated once again. Much that is importantly feminist was negated in this drama.

The Clinton scandal resonates because it authorized a political environment that was hostile to seeing a relationship between women's

138 humanity and their bodies, to seeing the impact of personal choices on larger communities. The masculinist political environs knot together with the economically racialized agendas of the medical complex. This contextual political setting defines the parameters in which breast cancer exists and is viewed.

The body as sex object and the body as medical health object are not one and the same, yet they are connected by a masculinist visor. So it mattered that President Clinton thought there were two kinds of women: the kind you fantasize fucking and the kind you marry. This is too traditionally classic to be interesting. However, he was the president of the u.s., so what he did or did not do mattered, and had effects not just at home. Bill groped Monica on the one hand and is married to Hillary on the other. He could not resist Monica even though he told us he tried. Those voluptuous full-rounded breasts and fleshiness were simply impossible to resist. Hillary was his intellectual partner; all brain, and not quite the right sexy body.

Gennifer Flowers, Paula Jones, Kathleen Willey, and Juanita Broaddrick all spoke of Bill's sexual, and sometimes unwanted, indiscretions. But the story is more complicated than simple sex. There were also Clinton's presidential appointments of Jocelyn Elders, Janet Reno, and Madeleine Albright. These women showed Bill's political commitment to gender equity in the public sphere. Gender equity means pretending there are no (sexual) bodies to contend with. Sexed bodies take us too uncomfortably into the personal and private realm. These women can be treated just like men. Bill's personal sexual politics was trumped by his public espousal of gender equity. He became unaccountable for his sexual exploits at the very moment they were exposed because they were said to be private.

The aftermath of sexgate was deeply troubling. The realm of bodily sex was reclaimed as personal and not political. Sexual harassment law by default was denuded of its political weight because unwanted sexual advances in the workplace were more readily viewed as simply personal rather than power-filled.[4] Women became their bodies all over again as Monica's weight and Linda Tripp's cosmetic surgery became the focus of late-night talk show jokes.

The radical feminist insight that our bodies are as political as they     139
are private was washed away in postsexgate rhetoric. In this washing the
complex relation between my individual choice about my body and the
power claims already written into and on it were rebifurcated. If my experience of sex harassment or domestic violence is my personal affair, so
is my exposure to carcinogens and to the masculinist constructs that occupy my body. This bifurcation relocates in strange places.

When the "personal is political," just how much of the personal is
political? What part of the personal is not political? Is the political personal in the same fashion that the personal is political? Liberal individualism begins with the notion of privacy and the division between politics
and the self. This becomes more true as the dominant discourse of neoliberalism—which emphasizes individual responsibility and favors corporate over government investment in formerly public domains—takes
hold. People think more of the self, less of the public; more of the personal, less of the political; more of self-help and less of governmental assistance; more of genes and less of environments.

In contrast, radical feminism in the late sixties brilliantly understood
that by starting with the self, its sexed bodily meaning, you could find
the political. One started with the self in order to find its structural constraints; one began with female bodies to uncover their gendered meanings; one began personally in order to act politically. Consciousness-
raising groups were initiated to create an understanding that the politicized meanings of womanhood could be found in individual lived experiences; or that by consciously uncovering one's own experience one
found the political ties constructing its meaning. Consciousness-raising
was meant not simply to find the self but to find the self as a part of
a larger political reality.[5] This place-consciousness becomes uniquely
subversive.

Radical feminism named and indicted the system of power as one of
sexual classes: men and women were in a class struggle with each other.
In its early viewings of this it lacked a conscious theorization of the
racial aspects of the sexual classes it exposed. By default, women and
their bodies were and remained white. Feminist women of color of
course knew more: that the self was also racially constructed.[6] When

140  race is denaturalized as white, then white skin is revealed as a privileged site, and whiteness becomes a color unto itself. Then one can name the silenced race-ing of sex and gender.

## How White Is the Personal?

Flesh has many hues of color. When flesh is thought to be white, it has already been defined by racialized power differences. White/caucasian is treated as the dominant flesh although it is a minority coloring across the globe. Breasts, like other body parts, are colored in this process. Dominant discourses constructed with this visor do not see different colors of flesh. Instead of seeing a mix of hues, a continuum of dark to light, a racialized whiteness is naturalized and silenced as such. Because no beginning point is recognized in this process of coloring, there is no recognition that the process of seeing is defined through power-differentiated lenses.

The privileging and domination of whiteness are established by a fixity of color.[7] The process of seeing or not seeing is enormously provocative in and of itself. Because we see with power meanings, the process of seeing or not seeing is already politicized before we look. Skin color has been given an inherent meaning that does not exist as such. Meaning is attached to color through the racialized and discriminatory visors of what race already means. Whiteness in its racialized form is given meanings that it does not innately have: goodness, intelligence, rationality, and so on.

Color represents racialized meaning in much the same way that gender represents the sexed body. If skin color is genetically determined, race is the cultural/political construction of its meaning; as sex is to gender. Sex and color are given their meaning through gender and race. Color matters only because its racial meaning makes it matter. Whereas any racial identification has a color, not every color is always seen accurately by its racial construction. So many mixed-race people are simply defined as black; or light-skinned blacks are defined as white; or my mother became negro because she was in a black hospital. Constructed settings make up color and with it race.

An antiracist feminism recognizes that once color and sex are denat- uralized as not simply biogenetic constructions, then breasts them- selves, as parts of female bodies, can be viewed as the environments they are, and house. This feminist *epistēmē* spotlights the cultural and politi- cal construction of bodies *and* pluralizes their individual variety.

## The Breast as White

The breast, in representing femininity, is simultaneously implicated in whiteness. The female body, despite its racial identity and multiplic- ity of colors, exists as a fantasized icon. The fantasy parades despite the many ways that reality negates it. Variety is displaced by singularity; col- ors become white. And, the white body becomes a universalized abstrac- tion: thin, large breasted, small waisted, with blond hair. If bodies are given imaginary status, pretense itself becomes naturalized. Anything can be pretended with breast augmentation, skin bleaching, hair dying, and so forth.

When historians of slavery look at the 1850s, they describe a "light- ening" and a "fusion" of colors. Slavery was not simply about blackness, because slavery was "becoming whiter." This lightening of color be- speaks the rape of black slave women by their white masters. Mulatto children often reveal this mixed-race history of slavery. They are a "walk- ing talking, breathing indictment of the world the white man made."[8]

Seeing colors is different from seeing black *or* white. The hues of honey, caramel, ivory, peaches-and-cream, mahogany, toffee, nutmeg, and so on bespeak a variety of colors and their histories. Such a mix of colors belies clear racial divides. It also becomes more difficult to use the abstract and universalized breast icon. It is not self-evident what white or black really means when at least 75 percent of african-ameri- cans are found to have at least one white ancestor.[9] Yet Lani Guinier, one of Clinton's abandoned nominees, was always referred to as black, although her mom is a white jew and her dad black.

This narrative is not just one of race but rather the racialized history of sex and its gendered meanings. This story is about racialized sex, the often-violent rape of slave women by their masters; about the race/gen-

142  dered humiliation and emasculation of slave men; about sex/race/gendered hatred and jealousy between slave-owner women and their female slaves.

This history is then also invested with the "purity" of white women who must be protected from racial mixing. White women's purity demands the protection of white women's sexuality. This control is keyly integral to the system of racialized patriarchy because white women construct the borders of racial differentiation. If white women are safe, then the race is safe, while white men are allowed their promiscuity, and black men are labeled predators.[10] Rodney King was continually beaten by the Los Angeles police long after he was down on the ground; Abner Louima was violently sexually assaulted by police officers in New York City after his arrest; forty-one bullets were shot at Amadou Diallo by the same police force for no apparent good reason. In each instance these men were simply seen as dangerous predators. In this context it does not really matter that the police officers saw Diallo pull a gun even though there was none. This deadly thinking sets the larger societal contexts in which breast cancer is whitened.

Sex is raced and race is sexual; gender is racialized and race gendered; there are colors to sexuality and sexualized colors, while colors are gendered as well. Bill Clinton is said to be almost black by Toni Morrison, calling attention to his positive affirmative action record: he appointed nearly half of all women and half of all black people who have ever served on the federal bench.

But Clinton also abandoned his appointees Johnetta Cole and Lani Guinier, both women of color, the minute right-wing criticisms were raised and the going got tough. Jocelyn Elders, also black, was dismissed as surgeon general as soon as she spoke publicly of masturbation as a necessary part of sex education for dealing with AIDS. One must also not forget Bill's ending of welfare as "we have known it," read by the public as ending the free ride for black women. The Clinton administration's contradictory civil rights politics expressed the new tensions among class, race, and sex in the global economy. On the one hand the globe is multiracial, while u.s. transnational capital remains predominantly white male.

It may seem that I have strayed a long way from the white breast, but not really. The white breast operates as a symbol of western-style femininity, which must be kept privileged, and therefore safe, in a larger world where most breasts are not white. It should not be lost on those of us living in the u.s. that Elizabeth Dole was a southern white woman running for the presidential nomination in 2000; and Hillary Clinton, who became a resident of New York in order to run for senator of New York, is identified with Arkansas.

Elizabeth Dole, as a white southern woman, spoke of family values with no child of her own and a husband who has become the poster boy for erectile dysfunction. One listened to her espouse the sanctity of our moral past and its traditional values, wondering whether this included slavery and the confederate flag. Meanwhile we were left to presume her sexless life, before Viagra, with Bob. This is a new kind of southern woman's purity.

On the other hand we have Hillary Clinton, also white and a little bit southern, also sexless compared with all of Bill's other women. She grew up in Park Ridge, a white suburb of Chicago, and was a Goldwater supporter in her youth. Her husband beds women, like the white master of old, even though the women we know of are white. But Hillary is still humiliated, like the white slave owner's wife who turns her head and pretends not to know. The personal is obviously political and also racialized to its core body. The task of white womanhood is to keep silent in exchange for its privilege. Too bad that this message is what the rest of the world received from the first lady of the u.s. as she traveled and was received across the globe.

## Feminism Impeached

If the personal is defined politically; and the breast is connected to the body and the body to its environs; and the political environs impact back on each layering; then it matters that the Clinton legacy says that the "personal is *not* political." This sets the larger context that disassociates the relational meanings of our bodies from their health. Part and parcel of these relations is the privatization of our communities and the

144 untrammeled growth of the private corporate sector. Clinton's presidency established the primacy of the globe over the nation, corporate over public needs, while declaring the personal as apolitical. Place-consciousness becomes divorced from the female body.

In August 1998 Bill Clinton finally succumbed and admitted an "inappropriate" relationship with Monica Lewinsky. After testifying for over four hours to the federal grand jury, he addressed the nation. He told us that the affair was wrong, that he had misled his wife, but then added: "It is private, it is nobody's business but ours. Even presidents have private lives."[11] He told us that he had never lied about any of this, and that it was not even sex, anyway.

More truthfully, all this is not just about sex. It is about sex and power differences. It is about power because sex *is* personal and private *and it is also* political. There was a difference between Clinton's personal and public life *and* there is *also* a politics to sex. One statement does not preclude the other.

Clinton maneuvered his way through the maze and avoided being impeached. Yet the whole story, as a national narrative, undermined years of feminist politics. Complexities about sex, sexual harassment, *and* the personal as political became horridly confused. Most media coverage of sexgate bungled the heart of the matter: that one's personal life is embedded in power relations, that bodies are never simply sexual/bodily and wholly private, that Clinton's gender/racial politics were better than his personal politics, *and* that he and Hillary had no right to enforce their kind of family on the rest of us. One can reject the sexual/racial moralism of a Ken Starr and the sexually puritan notion of promiscuity *and* still recognize that aspects of personal life are also politically consequential.

Because the personal is also always in part political, the body operates as much culturally as it does genetically. Given this, there is no sphere of safety that remains untouched by either the public or its environments. Yet the postsexgate narrative proclaims privacy for white men. Bill, and not Hillary, spoke of his indiscretions and asked for forgiveness. He chose privatization all the way around: from his sex life to corporate

agendas. Once-public arenas are replaced by private business and part-   145
nerships with government.

Clinton privatized the government and privatized the personal—
although the processes for doing so are not one and the same. Neoliberalism is in direct tension with feminism in this instance. It severs the relations between private and public life and throws individuals back on
themselves. In this climate there is little commitment to the public
health of women's bodies. It is ironic that Clinton was elected in 1992 on
the promise that he would solve the health care crisis. It just may be he
meant to solve the crisis in favor of pharmaceutical and drug companies, rather than for the rest of us.

Privacy, itself, has its own complicated history. It has no one charac-
terization given the racialized history of sex. Orlando Patterson believes
that african-americans stood by Clinton, even though he did so little for
them, because their own history has been "one long violation of their
privacy." Slavery denied all claims to privacy, allowing the slave owner
total power over the "slave's body and person." Even after slavery was
abolished, rights to privacy were continually violated. If the president of
the u.s. has no privacy, then what of them?[12]

The u.s. public was made to watch the entire drama of Bill, Hillary,
and Chelsea. The melodrama of their fractured family, featuring a dutiful even if angered wife, reminded women to stay put no matter how un-
happy or humiliated they might be in their marriage. Hillary's ratings
skyrocketed as she stood by her man and for her family.[13]  There has
been a slight shifting of familial rhetoric from "the family is a haven" to
"the family, even if broken, is better than nothing."

It is against this backdrop that Hillary ran for senator and Lizzie
Dole stumped for the Republican presidential nomination. One can
wonder whether it is a coincidence that women are allowed into the
electoral arena just as this public realm of government is being privatized and emptied of much of its power by global capital. So women
may now be welcomed into this arena as long as they mimic the traditional racialized and gendered format of dutiful wife.

Hillary told us that she was very committed to her marriage and

146 loved her husband and her daughter very much.[14] She is also often identified as a feminist icon of sorts. This simply confuses all the important issues like whose feminism is it anyway? Whose body? Whose privacy? Gwendolyn Mink asks which women Bill and Hillary care about and answers that it is white middle-class women who can afford family leave without pay, or who have the means to get an abortion, or who aspire to professional heights like the Cabinet. But poor mothers have been hurt by his welfare law, and women wage earners have been undermined by his treatment of women like Paula Jones.[15] As Maureen Dowd asks, did Hillary expect us to forgive Bill's "regressive private behavior with women" because of some of his "progressive public policies for women"?[16]

Clinton's personal secretary, a black woman named Betty Currie, was used by Bill as a go-between in the Lewinsky affair. I remember looking at Currie on t.v. as she was paraded to her first grand jury appearance, with terrified tension written all over her face. I thought how awful politics can be: our president has an older black woman for his personal secretary, and she becomes his liaison for his tryst with a white girl. She looks too much like the mammy slave with little choice. Race and sex are continually newly recombined in public fashion. Women's bodies are racially and culturally sculpted out of this old and new.

Antiracist feminists in the u.s. are the big losers in all this. Women elsewhere looked here and saw Hillary. Hillary went elsewhere and spoke her kind of western-style feminism. It is hard to create dialogues when the stakes are so high and there is so much distortion. At least sometimes there are diversions that are a bit of fun. Enter the women of the u.s. soccer team.

## Global Wars and Soccer Games

I want to refine the provocative understanding of "personal and political" without conflating them as one, *and* by seeing the political as both a racial and a sexual construction defined through class. Neoliberalism has forced a selfish politics on the globe. The self—its body, its breasts, its privacy—is disconnected and abstracted from the systems of

power defining it. Under this pressure, mainstreamed feminism has not
sufficiently held onto its radical moorings. Mainstreamed feminism
often stops with the self without speaking the power differences that impact women's bodies differently. Breast cancer activism also sometimes
suffers a selfishness when it presumes whiteness and western/middle-
class access to treatment.

The more the body is defined as simply private, the more politics is
left free to invade it. Gendered and racialized constructions of the female body, if not denaturalized, erase the tensions between sex and gender and between color and race. With no tension between them they
become effaced as one. Breast cancer cells then also become naturalized as genetically inherited or viewed as indicative of lifestyle choices
exactly when they must *also* be seen as a part of larger environmental
crises instigated by global capital.

Bodies are recontextualized out of the political relations that define
them. Radical feminists discovered the personal as political as they
fought against the Vietnam War. Thirty years later feminist theory was
written against the backdrop of the Gulf War. President Bush promised
it would be quick and easy, but the economic sanctions against iraq continue and Saddam Hussein remains in power. The war was an ecological disaster, and thousands of iraqi children continue to die of
malnutrition and disease as a result of u.s. policy. There was less media
exposure of rwanda's horrific war and pillage, but this did not make the
travesty of war less. The wars in bosnia and kosovo and chechnya have
been quieted but remain unresolved. Our government drops bombs instead of risking the bodies of our own troops.

Wars damage environments and the bodies that occupy them. Wars
redefine nations, and with this race and gender are renegotiated on the
globe.[17] This masculinist militarism functions even with many more
women in the military today than ever before. War rape in bosnia and
rwanda was part of this masculinist war machine. Women and children,
as civilians, died in great numbers in each of these wars. This contextual
backdrop of war and its destruction across the globe necessitates the
connection of breast cancer to these larger politicized environments.

The U.N. reported that the weeks of NATO bombing of iraq and

148    later kosovo destroyed the surrounding environments. In yugoslavia, land, air, rivers, and underground waters as well as the food chain were affected. Public water supply systems were incapacitated. There was damage to oil refineries, fuel dumps, and chemical and fertilizer factories. Toxic smoke from huge fires leaked harmful chemicals into the soil and water. Chemical pollutants like vinyl chloride and propylene filtered into the air. Many of the compounds released in these chemical accidents are known to cause cancer. Petrochemical spillage remains a part of the continuous bombing in iraq. All this is disastrous for ecological systems and people's health and women's breasts.

Breast tissue may be particularly susceptible to all this damage even if the connection is not as yet, understood. According to Sandra Steingraber, breast milk is now the most contaminated of all human food. She says that this is why a breast-fed infant has already received its so-called safe lifetime limit of dioxin in its first six months. "This milk, my milk, contains dioxins from old vinyl siding, discarded window blinds, junked toys" that have been incinerated and unleashed into the atmosphere. There is no question that these dangerous molecules are taken into the body and distilled in breast tissue and then into milk. So breast milk is dangerous and yet it is *also* a necessary assist for the infant's immune system.[18]

Steingraber sees women's bodies as the "first environment." Amniotic fluid, which is mainly composed of fetal urine, is made of what women drink and eat. It is made from the outside world and becomes the fetal environs. The only way to cleanse amniotic fluid of its impurities is to remove harmful chemicals and residues from "women's fat tissues, which means getting them out of the food chain, which means keeping them out of the environment in the first place."[19]

Political contextualization of women's bodies brings environmental constructions of them into complete view. Women absorb their environs, and their bodies are an environment for the fetus. These insights are smashed by masculinist warriors who victimize women by writing on their bodies with knives and bombs and war rape. Women's bodies absorb the political geographies of their local cultures. Women are stoned and punished by the Taliban in afghanistan, suffer honor killings for

alleged sexual promiscuity in jordan, and are victims of increasing in- 149
carceration in u.s. prisons. These environments cannot nurture
women's health.

Yet there is no one story line to tell here. Much also happens that
seemingly recognizes the importance of women in public life. Women
in kuwait may soon get the vote, lower-caste women (*panchayat*) have
been appointed to village councils in india, women are entering the
electoral arena in indonesia, women lead student strikes in iran, and u.s.
Secretary of State Madeleine Albright led the NATO bombing of serbia.
Women are taking their rightful place in public life; however, it is not
clear what this means for their private lives, their sexual selves, or their
bodily health. Nor does it say much about the daily lives of a great majority of women in each of these countries.

This becomes all the more complex in the u.s. with the corporatist
media attention on women's health issues and women's sports. The u.s.
women's soccer team won the 1999 World Cup, and there was much excitement about women's athleticism. Women's bodies are the focus of
this athleticism, but not passively as they are in porn. Strength and muscle matter for the physically fit woman. Brandi Chastain threw off her
jersey when she scored the winning kick. One sees her black athletic
bra, which holds her breasts tight and out of the way, and her muscled
arms. All the players are white except for Briana Scurry. Her black body
puts her color in clear view. The fantasized—flattened and not in clear
view—breast remains white.

These are women athletes, so breasts are not unimportant though
not prominent. The breast, whether visible or not, is fetishized by men
and women, even though this desire takes different form. Fixation with
the objectified breast motivates the Nike sports bra industry worth $250
million.

Women athletes encourage strong female bodies. Their bodies unsettle simple notions of femininity but not entirely. These athletes can
pluralize viewings of the female body. But more often than not, femininity is center-staged, and not displaced.

Soccer in the u.s. is touted as the suburban sport for preadolescent
and teenage girls. These girls are predominantly white and middle class.

150    Their moms are called soccer moms and are depicted as the hard working middle-class women of the new millennium. These moms were
considered the swing vote in the 1996 presidential election. After the
World Cup win, *Newsweek's* cover page read "Girls Rule." Interesting
choice of words given that almost all the players were in their thirties
and several were moms themselves. Maybe only girls are allowed these
bodies, and not women. Or maybe "Women Rule" is just too provocative.

Class and race and geographical location define the contours of this
spectacle. Those of us living in the u.s. should not allow ourselves to be
stunted by our immediate geographic space. As capitalism continues to
dominate the globe, the earth's resources become more endangered. As
long as a singular focus on profits defines corporate priorities, we shall
see more risk to the public's health. As bodies are assaulted by the effects
of war damage to the air and water, as chemical pollutants compromise
people's immune systems, as dietary habits shift as a result of global
transformations in agriculture, women will face new dangers.

The universalized breast allows for a partially shared reality of breast
cancer across the globe. And the specifics of different regions, nations,
and cultures also open up complex pluralities to investigate. Breast cancer, because it is more prevalent in westernized postindustrial societies,
should be seen as a warning sign for the rest of the globe. There may be
dietary and cultural practices in countries of the east and south for the
west to learn from. So we also need a global lens with localized clarity.

I still wish that Giah and Sarah were alive, that I could hear their
laugh, smell their presence, argue with them about whatever. But I
know that this can never happen. So I will settle for thinking about what
lets me feel close to them.

Breast health is a passionate place for thinking through to a "just"
world. It demands a kind of clarity of purpose that initiates seeing across
the divides of personal and political, local and global, hope and despair.

C  H  A  P  T  E  R  **S  E  V  E  N**

# Taking the Breast to the Globe

I AM CLEARING MY WAY FOR THINKING THROUGH to how a "really real" antiracist feminism needs to travel beyond itself. The traveling needs to be done *without* a staticized first- or third-worldization of women, which will allow for what I term *polyversal feminism*. *Poly-* means many or diverse. *Versal* is shorthand for designating the whole or entirety of a thing. Together they embrace the universality of humanity while demanding an earnest specifying of its different meanings; hence, *poly-* replaces *uni-*. This requires the deep belief that I can really learn and relearn from experiences that may not be my own.[1]

An antiracist feminism for 2000 must as Nawal El Saadawi says "unveil the mind," so that "really real" bodies can be seen.[2] I wish I could rid feminist dialogue of the western/nonwestern dichotomy so that we could move beyond oppositional mindsets that stunt our visioning. And

152   yet this wish is not completely doable because of the powerful authorization of the west by global capital and its version of democratic rights.

If antiracist feminist theory is the struggle to newly see, again and again, the emerging forms of sex/gendered racialization in order to challenge them, then we need to find the new faultlines of conflict over female bodies. In part we can see the Islamic fundamentalist attack on women—the Talibanization of women in afghanistan—as part of the same process which eliminates women peasant farmers in india. The process of economic globalization uncovers the patriarchal gendered priorities of the economic nation-state. The Taliban asserts its patriarchal identity against the homogenous rule of global capital while rural indian women are dismissed by corporate profiteers and the new urban middle class.

I am attempting to look globally without third-worldizing people in third-world countries; without glorifying and idealizing simplicity and noncorporatist farming; without homogenizing the west as a cyber/media capitalist monolith of power with nothing to offer, although *it* is often just this. Rather, an antiracist feminism must locate itself with the actuality of female bodies and their varieties and their varied geographical locations that are marked as sites through powered relations. Today, there are more instances of transnational feminisms as so many feminists of third-world countries live elsewhere than their homes. They wish to challenge the power of global capital by globalizing feminist solidarity for social justice.

Feminists cannot simply remain locally visioned. Although our geographical homes will play a part in developing new imaginings, the global contexts of these local experiences have keen impact.[3] The back and forth is complex because feminism's local sites are plural and their interactions with the global cannot be simply universalized. Because my local site is the u.s., I particularly must look elsewhere to find creative possibilities for negotiating and resisting its dominance. Because western-style individualism has its coordinates in a variety of other cultures, feminists in the west must know to look elsewhere to find new ways of opening up and radicalizing the meanings of individuality.

*Beyond Western Geography*

Let me unwind my thought more slowly here. Global capital is not located in any one geographical territory. When capitalism is described as "western," what domain is exactly referred to here? What is the "west"? West of what? If "west" today really refers to u.s. capitalism, then nonwestern influences and peoples inhabit this geographical territory with greater frequency than ever. I know their habitation does not displace the privileging of anglo-american culture. But I also hesitate to give even more endorsement to the power of the west by treating it hegemonically as u.s.-style democracy.

I also think that much of what is defined as western is *not* western, meaning capitalist, in its origin, but rather originates in many local geographies from what it means to be human. The belief that one's bodily entity is one's own to control and do with as one wills is borne within a variety of cultures, but is also linked to the polyversal realness of each of our individual bodies. Women claim their right to their body, or are unable to—against rape, forced pregnancy, prostitution—from within a polyversal belief that one's body is one's own.

Why identify this human claim of the right to one's body as western? Why give this claim to the west? Egyptian feminists in the early 1920s did not need to take claim to their bodily rights from anyone but themselves. African slave women did not need anyone but themselves to know that the stealing of their labor and their rape were actions deeply, horribly, against humanity. This claim to our bodies is what makes us human. It is not simply western, or equatable with bourgeois propriety or its derivative notion of individualism. One only has to look to see that the idea that one's body is one's own is written through a rich variety of cultural formulations because it is a site of consciousness.

Rosalind Petchesky argues along with her International Reproductive Rights Research Action Group (IRRRAG) that women's notion of owning their bodies has a transnational or translocal meaning in brazil, malaysia, mexico, nigeria, and the philippines, which cannot rightly be understood as simply western. Rather, bodily ownership is transversal

154 even if not expressed as a simply unity. She reveals the early work of the indian feminist and birth control advocate Kamaldevi Chattopadhyay, declaring woman's sacred right to control her own body, at the All-India Women's Congress in 1935.[4]

Starting with the body we find humanity, not the west. The site of universality—or polyversality—is our bodies. Our individual body's autonomy is established by its own demands, and not simply by the political language of western human rights which names these. This is as close as I want to get to a concept of the body as an authentic identity in and of itself. The seductiveness for today's women across the globe of human rights discourse derives from the consciousness of being human, because the body is the site for this political demand more than the western element of rights.

If I move away from the issue of sites of origin, I also wonder how one identifies an idea like feminism as western, when ideas travel and circle and overlap and dialogue. For women to wear lipstick in iran under the rule of Khomeini is not simply western; it is a statement of defiance that cannot easily fit within this oppositional categorization. So something is lost here if one is not looking to find the multiple sources and meanings in which to build an antiracist feminism for living across the globe.

When women in islamic countries defy interpretations of the shaaria that they know to be unjust, when women in cuba demand lesbian rights, when women in nigeria lead the movements against environmental degradation, when women in pakistan, and india, and south africa demand better medical access for dealing with breast cancer, they are all speaking from their localized bodies and their cultural meanings that voice a shared experience across the globe. The pull and seductiveness of feminism derive from the truths of bodily experiences. Western-style capitalism exploits as well as reveals the body, while more and more "of and from the body" is marketed for sale. One should not confuse this unveiling of the body as one and the same with universal rights or democracy.

If western stands in for the notion of "colonized bodies," this cuts both ways and several ways and the west is no longer a place, if it ever was. It is a set of ideas that navigates and travels everywhere. But as a hegemonic force it also colonizes the multiplicity of meanings that are not simply west, nor simply local. And yet if I am going to be politically honest I must deal with the power differentials that are real, even if not always true, between west *and* nonwest. I must recognize the divide, and acknowledge it. But I must also insist on intellectually and politically unsettling the meaning of "west." This is a demanding process that takes time and requires enormous generosity of people whatever space they inhabit.

Women from india living in the u.s., women from iran living in Amsterdam, women from egypt living elsewhere and sometimes locating at home are part of the similar processes that market teriyaki burgers in japan, tacos in Harlem, thai food in most u.s. big cities. Gastronomic pluralism is simply that and something much more; a beginning process of cultural/local/global mixing.[5] Local identities are not irrelevant, and yet they do not have a static original meaning when we see women running cybercafés in Cairo and others on motorbikes with their saris flying in Delhi, or signs for women's workout gyms outside of Accra.

All this said, it is also the case that the promissory tension of bourgeois individualism—that achievement rather than ascription is open to anyone—is translocally a politically compelling and formative vision. This powerful notion is translated when specific cultural meanings already wait to be discovered. However, the local discovery is not only a reactive or colonial process but rather it is a dialogic interplay that is not singularly oppressive. So there is much to be learned from these political processes of discovery and re-vision. The claims to individuality do not remain western-capitalist even if the claims *sometimes* begin through this route.

## Glocal Phallusies and the "Really Real"

The mix that I term *glocal* can reveal several liberatory meanings of feminism that are not understood best as existing because of the west, or

156  from the west, but rather may be understood in relationship with the west.[6] But west is better termed global-west, because then it becomes situated as power-filled rather than as a singular location.

New forms of colonialism are written by cyberculture's supposed global village, which denies much of the world access to communication. Transnational capital dominates world economies, while more and more communities inside the u.s. are dominated. Islamic fundamentalists target "their" women for strict controls against the influences of the west. And the global media corporations target these fundamentalists while covering over patriarchal abuses in the global-west.

Seeing and naming change *within* the systems of power are subversive of the discourses that congeal power systems. The trouble here can be *both* those who are interested in protecting systems of power and those who are interested in changing and dismantling these systems. Those committed to change are often invested in language that is no longer *really* helpful in revealing new complexities and their opportunities for change.

Today, the cybervirtual real and the media-fantasy real complicate and distort ways of knowing, seeing, and naming. The distortion is newly wired through the very old systems of race and gender, nation and globe. Seeing is more plural and interwoven than the process of naming readily allows for. Hence the homogenized categories that populate our viewing: black/white; woman/man; biogenetics/environment; women of color/white women; west/nonwest.

Racialized gender is always in the process of construction, changing along with the contexts of the moment, yet language is less fluid, and gets stuck, and we are unable to see, name, and act on it. Reality has become more real *and* unreal, fantasy, and virtual. There are few clear markers of the "fantasy real," and yet they must be unveiled. In looking for them I move as carefully as I can with my own invested blinders to try and name the glocal phallusies that inhibit "really real" knowledge.

For me, nationalism is a fantasized imaginary that maps political geography on women's bodies, while also erasing the process of doing so. Globalism, also fantasized, is part of this renewed erasure at the millennium. Meanwhile women compose 70 percent of the world's 1.3 billion

poor, and one-half of Africa's population, about 300 million people, live
without access to basic health care.[7] In tanzania where 40 percent of the
population dies before the age of thirty-five, the government must spend
nine times more on foreign debt payments than on health care.[8] In the
u.s. over 108 million lack dental insurance, and a "silent epidemic of
oral diseases" is affecting its poorest citizens.[9] African women account
for close to 80 percent of women infected with AIDS worldwide yet
Africa accounts for just 1 percent of world drug sales.[10] Africa suffers its
millions of AIDS orphans, while billions are spent elsewhere by corporations on averting Y2K computer disruption. Meanwhile there is no
lack of new drugs for hair loss and obesity in rich nations, while people
living in poverty go without necessary nutrition and treatments for diseases like malaria and cholera.

Forty percent of the globe has no electricity, and 70 percent of the
earth's people have never made a phone call. In india 0.5 percent of
households have internet access, telephone lines are installed before toi-
lets and latrines in places like haiti and cambodia, while still more than
half of the world population lives more than two hours from a telephone. According to a U.N. development study there is approximately
one internet user per every 1,200 people in Africa, one in every 125,000
in Latin America and the Caribbean, one in 250,000 in East Asia, one in
500,000 in the Arab states, and one in 25,000 in South Asia.[11] Instead of
creating a global village, new hierarchies are formed with all of these
technologies. A racialized gender politics emerges as family, nation, and
globe are renegotiated.

National governments are no longer able to curtail global capital,
while commitments to public life are downsized and smothered. The
International Monetary Fund orchestrates the privatization of every possible space, while racialized patriarchy runs rampant across women's
bodies. So transnational corporations restructure nation-states, and
racialized patriarchy is reconstituted along with the nation-state. Once
again feminisms must relocate themselves within and against these
transformations.

This is the backdrop against which I traveled to cuba, canada, and
ghana. My locale and my commitment to seeing beyond it frame my ex-

158 periences and my understanding of them. I wished to discover new ways of understanding how environmental contexts influence and impact the health of women and girls as well as the rest of the globe. More specifically, I wondered if breast cancer translates across cultures as a rallying point for women as it does in the u.s. or whether poverty, and AIDS, and maternal mortality, and malaria set a more complicated context that both enriches and demands polydimensional approaches. I am still wondering how breast cancer activism—which is so passionately adopted—can better assist women's activist struggles as a place of resistance, to reclaim social justice for the people of the globe.

## My Traveling to Cuba

In April 1998 I was part of the u.s. MADRE delegation to the International Women's Conference in Havana. MADRE is an international women's human rights organization. Approximately three thousand women from seventy-six different countries from all continents met here. My delegation brought with it approximately a $250,000 worth of donated medicines. I had collected sixty pounds of birth control pills, antibiotics, and children's medicines from doctors in my community.

For several weeks before leaving for cuba my daughter and Richard helped me punch the pills out of their Styrofoam wraps so that I could sort them more compactly and fit more into each carton for easy transport. When we were done we were left with five huge bags of Styrofoam garbage to dispose of. I couldn't help thinking that the packaging was stupidly excessive and wasteful.

The time in cuba made me more conscious than ever of the oppressive effects of "my" government on other countries. The conference was filled with women from all parts of the world who were committed to helping cuba against the u.s. embargo. I would walk to the conference hall from my hotel, through incredible poverty but also vibrancy. As a tourist, I was fed well, provided with bottled water, and negotiated the two economies—local and global—existing side by side. Outside the hotel there were always two different kinds of cabs waiting. One was a tourist cab, meaning you paid in dollars and it was relatively expensive. The other was a "local" cab, based on the peso, and very inexpensive.

As I walked, every bike that passed me had as many people on it as it    159
could possibly provide. The medical clinics I visited were quite amazing
despite their clear need for more supplies of every sort and kind. The
AIDS sanatorium I visited made me think that if one were poor in the
u.s., one would definitely do better for treatment here in cuba. I was
deeply impressed with the way cuba utilizes its limited resources.

I was also conscious of the clearly gendered workforce in the medical clinics I visited. Men held the leadership and authority positions in
almost all. I also got tired of being eyed and spoken to by so many of the
boys and men who would pass me on the street and think they could say
whatever they wished. The banter did not feel friendly, but aggressive. I
would feel annoyed, wonder if it was because I was a hateful yankee, or
just because I was a woman. Whatever the reason, I was conscious of a
difference that I did not like.

I left cuba thinking a lot about its poverty, its incredible resilience
on the medical front, and the enormous generosity of the women I met
despite what felt like a masculinist culture to me. I also thought that as
an outsider I did not fully know how these women felt as insiders,
whether they found the machismo constraining in their own ways, and I
was left wanting to better understand my own experience as an outsider
from the u.s.

My head was filled with these thoughts as I left Havana and headed
home. Then, while I was waiting for a connecting flight in the Philadelphia airport, CNN announced the death of Linda McCartney. She had
died of breast cancer despite the incredible medical care available to
her. I thought, again, as always, about Sarah and Giah.

I felt sad and alone, the way one can feel in an airport. I sat and felt
the relentlessness of breast cancer, the way it sometimes makes you feel
vulnerable all over again. And I also thought how unjust it is that the u.s.
embargo against cuba makes it almost impossible for women to get the
preventive care and treatment for breast cancer they need, and how u.s.
politics toward cuba and the economic crises it creates have assisted in the
renewal of sex tourism and prostitution for women there. It felt hateful.

Women in the u.s. need to know that the embargo and its wide rang-
ing effects mean more black and brown women will die from breast cancer in cuba than need to. The effects of the embargo mean that early

160    detection and treatment are increasingly unavailable. Until 1990, mammograms were available at no cost to all cuban women over thirty-five.[12] Today only women who are considered at high risk can get mammograms. Although mammograms are no panacea, they remain the only chance some women have for early diagnosis.

    The embargo has undermined the entire system of universal health care that exists in cuba. Signs are up throughout Havana demanding that the u.s. be humanitarian and stop the embargo. I flinched each time I saw these signs; as I did in the conference hall each time Castro blasted the u.s. for its blockade and we joined other women in the convention hall chanting: "Cuba Si! Bloques no!"

    According to "A 1977 Report from the American Association for World Health," cuba has two mammogram units based at medical institutions in Havana and fifteen mobile units. Each unit can perform some four hundred mammograms per week. By 1994 and 1995, owing to lack of x-ray film, there were regional shut-downs of the screening process. The embargo prevents Eastman Kodak—a main maker and distributor of X-ray film—from selling its film to cuba.[13]

    Owing to the lack of surgical supplies, many women cannot have the breast-related surgeries they need. Women wait for months for limited treatments. The u.s. dominance of the cancer drug market means that many breast cancer therapies are unavailable to cuban women. Because approximately 80 percent of all medical drugs worldwide are produced by u.s. companies or their subsidiaries, cuban women are denied access to the drugs that could possibly save their lives. This is still most often the case even though there have been some recent modifications of the embargo to allow for medical supplies.

    This is why MADRE initiated the "Share Hope Campaign" in 2000 to assist in the donation and delivery of tamoxifen—to be used for treatment but not for preventive purposes—to the Red Cross in cuba. This began MADRE's two-year effort to bring intensive support to the women of cuba in their struggle to survive breast cancer.

    Breast cancer takes too many lives, even with the best medical care available. It is a moral outrage to have to face it under the terms of an embargoed economy that denies women a fighting chance to try to stay

alive. At least Linda McCartney had every imaginable treatment available to her. It is heartbreaking that this was not enough to save her life,
but at least she was able to try. What about women in cuba who will die,
not because they have breast cancer, but because they do not have access to any mode of early detection, or because chemotherapy drugs that
might save their lives are embargoed or just too expensive for a country
living under the effects of an embargo? The economic and political environs that engulf these women are clearly as deadly as any cancer gene.

My outrage brings me back to my own locale where poor women in
the u.s. who have no medical insurance to pay for mammograms do not
get them, or women who live in rural communities where there is no
easy access to medical facilities cannot be screened. Some deaths from
breast cancer at this moment cannot be deterred, but some can. This is
why breast cancer activism must continue to enlarge its umbrella to
women across racialized class lines in the u.s. and across the globe.

It is amazing to read of Jeri Nielsen, a doctor "trapped" in the South
Pole at the Amundsen-Scott research station until the October thaw
with a lump in her breast. An Air Force jet dropped medical supplies for
her needed diagnosis and treatment. With the so-called thaw a cargo
plane with a ten-man crew swooped down in sixty-degree below zero
weather to bring her home. If only every woman could be assured a little bit of such attention.[14]

## Glocal Politics at the Ottawa World Breast Cancer Conference

I went to the Second World Conference on Breast Cancer to deliver
a plenary talk that would criticize the dominant-western privileged dialogues constructing and surrounding breast cancer.[15] Here is a perfect
instance in which I am still bounded by the necessity and limitations of
the category "the west."

I was in the process of writing this book when I went. Sarah came
with me. It would be the first time I would speak from the book, and I
was comforted by her company.

I also went to Ottawa because I wanted to participate in the radical-
ization of u.s. breast cancer activism as it moves from the u.s. to other

162 parts of the globe. And I wanted to see how the narratives and activism in other countries could enlarge my understanding of my local site.

When I arrived in Ottawa, although it was advertised as a world conference it felt less so. The corporate sponsorships probably added to my sense of this as western, and western bespeaks globalism to me more than the world. Materials and advertisements displaying information on the latest breast cancer techniques and treatments bespoke the priorities of the medical establishment more than progressive activism. Medical treatments like lumpectomy, breast reconstruction, and tamoxifen were privileged in most of the literature distributed. Although this was just one presence at the conference, it was the dominant one.

I call attention to the corporate sponsorship of the conference not to condemn the organizers but rather to highlight the incredible pressures and constraints impacting on breast cancer activism. One needs money to host a conference; just as one must have funding to do one's research. So in this monied setting, of course there will be complicity and compromise. Therefore activists must push out the limits as far as they can to limit the damage.

After the morning session, I walked into the ballroom filled with circular tables set up for small group discussion. I was most interested in talking to African doctors and activists because I especially was wondering how the whiteness of the western breast translates there. I looked for name tags and walked toward a table filled with people from senegal, india, and ghana, and sat down.

My first conversation was with a doctor Papa Coure from Dakar, senegal. I asked him which surgical procedures he used most frequently, and he answered that he most often, almost 80 percent of the time, performed mastectomies. I asked why, and realized later that I had thought I already knew the answer: that there was a lag from here to there in the latest treatments and techniques. But this was not the case at all. The reason he performed mastectomies was quite simply that almost all the cases he sees are diagnosed at very late stages. He himself had been trained to do surgical lumpectomy at Sloan-Kettering.

Although he has used chemotherapy to shrink large tumors and then perform lumpectomies, this is very rarely possible because most

women cannot afford this protocol. As well, there are few centers that   163
can provide the follow-up radiation necessary for postlumpectomy treatment. Doctor Coure made clear that poverty and the lack of access it
creates greatly inhibit the treatment of breast cancer in senegal. Trained
in the west, he still is unable to share the variety of treatments available
in the u.s.

Much of the discussions in which I partook were about the lack of
access to treatment protocols, as well as medicines and breast prostheses.
Several women from india and pakistan spoke about the problem of self-
image for women facing breast cancer. They said that many of the
women they dealt with ignored early signs of disease because they could
not bear the thought that they would lose a breast. One woman from the
Delhi branch of Cancer Sahyog, an emotional support group for people
living with cancer and their families, told me how very many of the
women who had had mastectomies refused to leave their homes. She
said that if only good prostheses could be made available to them, their
lives would greatly improve. Prostheses in india are made of rubber, are
too lightweight and flimsy, and most women even if they can afford
them won't wear them.

While listening, I remember thinking how incredibly fast the self-
help, self-esteem language of the western breast cancer movement had
traveled to other parts of the globe, to women from so many different
places. So much of the talk I was hearing related to women's body
image, sense of self-worth, and preciousness of the breast. I was taken
aback. I thought, I have gone to a world conference, and met the west
from everywhere. I kept mulling this over and thought: maybe this love
and fear of the body is not the west. Maybe it is the body speaking the
self in transnational and polyversal ways across enormous cultural divides. If there is a starting point, it is the body speaking itself.

It was at the Ottawa conference that I consciously began to move my
thinking in this direction. I now was listening differently, more openly,
with less sense that I already knew what I thought. I realized that many
of the concerns being shared have their own local bodily meaning that
cannot simply be described by identities like west or nonwest. Women's
fear of breast cancer is homegrown within their bodies along with their

164   bodies' specific cultural meaning. This is a complicated knotting of their geographical context and the locally specific beliefs and traditions through which loss of a breast gets translated. *And* this mechanism is also incredibly similar to the one that creates an idealized symbolic woman's body—from consumerist visions of the rock star Madonna to the idealized indian goddess Devi. There is something very localized yet global here. So, yes, the global-west is not irrelevant, but it tells only a piece of the story.

In sudan rural women have little access to information or services; in india there are too few detection centers and little availability of treatment except in big cities; in myanmar mammography is not yet feasible for routine screening; in kenya breast cancer is the leading cause of death for women between thirty-five and fifty years of age. Women in nigeria say they need much more to be done about detecting breast cancer in the first place. In romania the incidence of breast cancer mortality is high and growing. In puerto rico most breast cancer detection is at the later stages of disease, which has become a major cause of death for women older than fifty.

The conference focused more on detection and treatments than on prevention strategies. Most of the informal discussions I partook in were similarly occupied. Many speakers spoke from the dominant medical and/or environmental discourses with little radical intervention into their political pre-suppositions. There was much focus on the risk factors defining the global incidence of breast cancer and the necessity of trying to limit new risk.

A clear exception to this prevalent discourse was Andaiye, from guyana, who delivered an address titled "Cancer and Power." She began by confessing that her presentation "arises out of rage, since my whole experience of having cancer (non-Hodgkin's 1989–91) and of being a cancer activist in one small, poor country has been and is a battle with and against powerlessness." She declared that the greatest risk factor facing women living in third-world poor countries was living in a third-world country. Andaiye argued that powerlessness to change the "national inequalities" that force people to inhabit unsafe/unhealthy environments *is* the leading cause of cancer today. She relocated risk factors away from one's particular genetic body, to one's political, geographic, and economic environments.

Andaiye argued that if women are too poor to adequately prevent their exposure to environmental risks, how does it even make sense to discuss treatment, which is out of reach for most women anyway. She refused to start anywhere other than at the beginning of the problem, which for her is at the point where "power hierarchies of gender, race/ethnicity, class and nation intersect."[16]

The many men and women from different continents, dealing with one disease that most probably is not completely singular to begin with, allowed for an uncomfortable dialogue about who gets to define disease, and its prevention, and its treatment. The powerful relations constructing breast cancer—its research, its prevention, its treatments—are as *real* as it gets because they define who is going to have a fighting chance against death on this planet.

So I went to Ottawa to critique the western biases imbricated inside breast cancer and to learn of possible new ways to be able to do this. I learned that the west as a construct does not let me see *some* of the connections which exist between women across the west/nonwest divide. And I realized that some of the focus on personal body image is hardly just western. Many of the women I met and spoke with from india, ghana, and indonesia were incredibly similar to many of the breast cancer activists in the u.s in the way they thought of their bodies and breasts. In part this may simply be indicative of who primarily attends a conference of this sort to begin with. But, at least in part, this conference dialogue also bespoke the rich intersections between bodies and their environments. These overlaps allow for translocal connection and glocal learning.

On the other hand I was also reminded, especially by Andaiye's talk, that the global-west cripples poor nations and smothers their people's chances for a healthful life. In other words, bodies are always environmentally contextual no matter how seemingly similar. I think my notion of polyversal begins to capture the tension between these two sites: the body's sameness and its particularized meanings.

On the drive home from Ottawa, Sarah told me she thought it was

166  good that I did not wear my prostheses when I gave my talk. She said no one could tell, anyway.

### Speaking in Ghana with the Globe

I had never been to Africa before, and I wasn't really going to Africa, because I was just traveling to Accra, ghana. Sarah and Richard went with me. They said I could not leave them out of this new experience. After arriving at the airport we drove through lush green countryside filled with people working along the roadside and in the fields. We saw women carrying and selling foodstuffs on their way to market. We saw a country starkly different from our own. Sarah just kept looking out the window. Her first words were that she maybe now knew a little what it felt like to be a black at her school. It took her a few days to stop hating her whiteness because it would not let her blend in.

I spoke at the "Women and Earth" conference just as the year 2000 was to begin. I would share my thoughts about the effects of global capitalism on women and girls. I was completely conscious of speaking from the u.s., and as a white woman in a sea of black and brown faces. It took me back to my days in Atlanta. But in Accra I knew what I wanted to try and do.

I started to speak. "It is a daunting task to clear the space from which we can hear and see one another, across our power-filled differences, through our invested visors, in between the locations of displacement, fear, and hope. As a woman with the white skin of the ashkenazi jew, living in the u.s., this is not completely possible, and yet I will push as hard as I can to do so."

I ask the women and men attending the conference—from england, nigeria, the u.s., iran, ghana, australia, rwanda, and so on—to try and really think and theorize along with me; I tell them that the theory is necessary in order to try and really see. And really seeing means being able to grasp the ways moments and their structures of power change while language and naming often occlude and mystify. I then unpack my understanding of the *structures* of transnational capitalist racialized patriarchy in the cybermedia corporate global economy.

Instead of a "new world order," I expose the chaos of nationalist wars 167
and global exploitation. In the hopes of building toward an antiracist/
colonialist feminism for the millennium, I explore the difficulties posed
for women and girls across the globe as we face new-old forms of racialized patriarchy operating at the behest of transnational capital.

Because the globe is *not* a village; because the powerful monocul-
ture of transnational capital makes it so hard to speak, or see, or hear
each other, inside the nation, or across and beyond it/them; because the
environment is being degraded along with our bodies, I travel to the cy-
berenvirons of the filthy rich back to the contaminated breasts and
breast milk of women of all colors. I ask the audience to really think despite the "real fakes" of the cyberglobe.

I meet the west in ghana too, but "west" here means an embrace of
the cybereconomy of global capital. Many of the people I spoke with
were eager to find ways to create access to better jobs and education for
women in their communities. One professor at a university just outside
Accra was involved in an outreach project to teach rural women how to
use computers. Several women from iran spoke of the importance of
opening more opportunities in education. Others spoke of the significance of electoral politics. There was little critique of the structural requisites of global capital and more concern with bringing women into
the economy on an equal footing. Western consumer culture has a lure
all of its own.

In my discussion I emphasize the crisis facing women today due to
the privatization of the earth's resources and its people, with especially
grave consequences for women and girls. I name capitalist racialized patriarchy, not capitalism, as the universalized system, and the naming is
significant so it can be *seen* as such. This theorization allows for a historical memory tied to a present that is power-filled.

I continue and try to pluralize my examples from distant parts of the
globe. The obscene levels of profits for the rich and upper classes obscure the particular ways that race and gender are exploited by multicul-
tural corporatism and the exported forms of westernized feminism.[17]
These are new forms of corruption that both destabilize and recode
women's and girls lives. One should also not mistake feminism for

168   export as one and the same as feminisms of and in the west which are more multiple and complex given the many identities of women in any location.

Similarly, we need to see the complexities of islamic feminists and their struggles within religious fundamentalist regimes. Islamic feminists, often seen simply as dupes of the west, are misunderstood in their specific struggles both inside and outside the nations in which they live. The imagery of women in islam has become a symbolic export for global consumption, a new faultline of struggle between nationalisms that are inherently patriarchal *and* global capital's smashing of statist patriarchal controls. Women in islam, in spite of and because of their variety, have initiated some of the crossfire and are also caught within it.

As well, postcommunist feminists throughout Eastern Europe now suffer the consequences of their various revolutions of 1989. Their commitment to nonpatriarchal democratic regimes has been tempered by the harsh realities of their new market economies. Women in russia, bulgaria, the czech republic, and so on have lost their jobs *and* the state supports of old. The economies work mainly for transnational capital and the thugs it creates. Majorities in bulgaria, russia, and poland say that what they have gotten is not what they wanted or expected. Women beggars are common, alongside porn and prostitution. Given all this, it is almost impossible to reclaim the democratic imaginary for feminism. And many women in eastern europe are not sure that the language of feminism is sufficient for their needs anyway.

Women's struggles in algeria, south africa, and nigeria present enormous variety. Women struggle against the violence of their political regimes as well as the violence in their private lives, the degradation of the poverty created by the policies of the IMF and World Bank, and famine, and *yet* build communities of women out of this that also express self-determination for themselves and their countries. The United Nations offers an assist in this direction with its multiple initiatives that are women-focused. Although sometimes U.N. initiatives are simply forms of imperialist feminism, more often than not they initiate important opportunities. The U.N.'s women's agenda is complex and variable. In part, it is a politics articulated by women themselves and therefore not simply western because this transnational activism is no longer

solely of the west. Feminism's home turf is the women, and their female   169
bodies, that travel across and through these multiple geographical and
cultural locations.

Racialized patriarchy is transnational and experienced through
polyversal female bodies. So the language of west/nonwest, north/south,
first world/third world, global/national, *and* biogenetics/environs, na-
ture/culture, and personal/political must be thought through *through*
these divides. These divisions though real and with consequence are
also not *simply* divides. They connect transnational structures of power
with women and girl's lives while also recognizing cultural and economic class distinctions. Racialized patriarchy has "glocalized" meanings that women and girls must really try to see. The seeing is not easy
because the relations of power exist in part to obscure vision.

Consumer culture presents images and visual screenings that are
never either wholly false or completely true. Bare breasts, veils, lipstick,
chadors, blue jeans, porn, sati, henna, nose rings, and spike heels each
have their many meanings. Each practice is intimate *and* public. Deep
red lipstick *can* be an act of defiance in iran, and simple consumer culture in New York City or Bangkok . . . and neither. And the markets in
Accra are filled with local foodstuffs, and as much plasticized junk made
in thailand and the philippines as you can possibly imagine, as an em-
blem of western global consumerism.

Before leaving ghana I spoke with women about the shame they felt
about their breast cancer, and how some had found their husbands de-
spondent about their disease, and how they turned away from them. But
breast cancer is not spoken easily and its presence is much lower in
Africa than in other parts of the world; 10–20 per 100,000 people. But
when I shared this statistic with one woman, she asked me how anyone
*really* knows what the rate of breast disease is. She wanted to know
which communities in Africa they studied for the statistics.

On our last day in ghana we went to Elmina Castle. This is where
slaves were kept before their passage to america. Sarah stood next to me
in the courtyard with the sign "female slaves" overhead, and we held
each other's hand as an incredibly articulate guide told their story. Sarah
says she will never forget being there. I don't think she will.

*"Really Real" Feminism*

Women and girls across the globe, many of whom live in diasporic communities, are confronted daily with the disastrous effects of global capital. Food and agricultural systems are being corporatized, creating new levels of ecological and health hazard. This corporatization displaces indigenous people, many of them women, who have sustained and maintained the biodiversity of food and plants. Activists like Vandana Shiva warn against the biotechnology and agrichemical corporations that violate nature-friendly ecological sustainability. Activists meeting at the Solidarity Convention of People against Globalization, held in New Delhi in March 2000, demand the securing of healthful food, a clean environment, and an end to polarizing inequalities and economic injustices.

There are new levels of poverty, especially for women and girls; new crises of the environment and public/global health; the continuation of diseases like TB and malaria and especially AIDS; the daily suffering too often ignored caused by chronic reproductive tract infections, as well as continuing high rates of maternal mortality; and maybe the spread of breast cancer to the poorest sites of the globe where wastes are dumped and water is polluted.[18]

As long as profit rather than health defines corporate priorities, we shall see more breast cancer across the globe because it is an effect of global capital's arrogance. As bodies are assaulted by the effects of war damage to the air and water, as chemical pollutants compromise people's immune systems, as dietary habits shift as part of global transformations in agriculture, women will face new breast cancers. Breast cancer, more prevalent in postindustrial countries of the west should be seen in part as a warning sign for the rest of the globe. And the late diagnosis of breast cancers in senegal, ghana, and other poor countries bespeaks another warning: that excessive poverty in African nations charts a different breast cancer scenario where mammograms, and radiation, and chemotherapies are beyond the reach of most women.

This is not to mention the difficulties for women with breast cancer living under the economic sanctions in iraq. Or of women in cuba living under the constraints of the u.s. embargo. The transnational/u.s. corporate *glocal* dominance of the cancer drug market means that many breast cancer therapies remain unavailable to women without means everywhere.

Contaminated breasts are a telling warning sign. According to Sandra Steingraber breast milk is about "10 to 100 times more contaminated with dioxins than the next highest level of stuff on the human food chain." This is why a breast-fed infant has already received its supposed "safe" lifetime limit of dioxin.[19]

However, a woman needs enough caloric intake to make breast milk in the first place. Excessive poverty affects women's breast milk and therefore their new infants. No milk or watered-down milk causes early malnutrition and unnecessary suffering. For AIDS-infected women, breast milk is a danger to their infants, but infant formula is very often too expensive. Infant formula is most often an inadequate replacement for breast milk and is also useless without a safe water supply. Then, again, who wants dioxin-laced breast milk. These are unacceptable choices for the women and people of the globe.

I am almost back to where I started. The body is always personal and also political; always local and also global; always distinct and also shared; always sexed and colored *and* also gendered and raced; always genetic and also environmental; always glocal and potentially feminist. As such, the body is an incredible place to build resistant consciousness.

## Justice for the Breast

I know that my journey has traveled a strange path with maybe unexpected turns and unclear directions. I start with the breast but then argue that it is always already something else besides itself, that it is tied to its environments through power-filled relationships.

The *real* despair of breast cancer is too compelling not to use toward developing an activism for a truly just democratic globe. Please do not read this as some sort of essentialist plea that reduces women to their bodies, or their misery. Instead I write from my body which is no longer simply female in order to move us beyond a singular site of loss. Frida

172 Kahlo, the mexican artist, drew from her pain-ridden body to create "infinite variety" rather than "stale sickness."[20] Rachel Carson finished writing her pathbreaking defense of the environment, *Silent Spring,* while dying from breast cancer. Audre Lorde used her breast cancer as a visor to dig deeply into and against the power systems of her life.

Let this politics from the breast reject the excesses of greed that destroy the earth and our bodies with it. Feminisms across this globe must say no to the transnational corporate agenda that pollutes our bodies, steals labor, ruins the air and soil and streams, smashes the varieties of rich cultural pleasure, and leaves too many with too little. In reclaiming our bodies as a subversive *place,* especially in this cybereconomy, we can construct an intimate and passionate politics for the millennium. This *really* democratic imagining becomes a site from which a "really real" democracy can be written.

We must take our breasts with us, whether they are a body part or not, and begin again and again to build new notions of glocal democracies that are enriched by the polyversality of our bodies. The breast, with its diverse potentials—maternal, sensual and sexual, heartfelt, polluted, and objectified—remains an unstable and therefore promissory site for transnational or polyversal feminisms.

Governance from this site is our best hope for a world that will never see yellow stars, or pink triangles, or slave ships filled with black and brown bodies, again. In this world, disease prevention will be the only way corporations can make money. Health screenings and detection services will be available free of charge. Treatments will be available to all who need them. Healthy bodies will be a human right. And maybe in this world we will no longer need either pink or red ribbons.

I know that Sarah and Giah would be fighting for this world if they were alive.

# NOTES

## One. Familial Breast Cancer Bodies

1. As in my previous books, I do not capitalize countries, to call attention to their transnational status in a global capitalist patriarchal economy. I also do not capitalize racial/ethnic identities, in order to challenge their static and exclusive meanings. Instead, I wish to see the fluid and changing meanings of both national and racial identification. This stance also affects my understanding of breast cancer's construction.

2. Several writers assisted me in this process of writing my pain. See Louise de Salvo, *Breathless: An Asthma Journal* (Boston: Beacon Press, 1997); Mark Doty, *Heaven's Coast: A Memoir* (New York: HarperCollins, 1996); and Joan Nestle, *A Fragile Union: New and Selected Writings* (San Francisco: Cleis Press, 1998).

3. Arthur Laurents, *Original Story By: A Memoir of Broadway and Hollywood* (New York: Alfred A. Knopf, 2000), 234.

4. Audre Lorde, *The Cancer Journals* (Argyle, N.Y.: Spinsters Ink, 1980).

## Two. My Other Bodies

1. I am indebted to Grace Lee Boggs for the notion of "place-consciousness," in her "A Question of Place," *Monthly Review* 52, no. 2 (June 2000): 19. Although she does not use the phrase to elaborate a body-consciousness, we share a similar commitment to the importance of local sites for political action against global indifference.

2. Luce Irigaray, *This Sex Which Is Not One* (Ithaca: Cornell University Press, 1985). Also see Elaine Marks and Isabelle de Courtivron, eds., *New French Feminisms: An Anthology* (Amherst: University of Massachusetts Press, 1980).

3. Of course there are many feminists who deal specifically with the body, like Simone de Beauvoir, Luce Irigaray, Hélène Cixous, Marguerite Duras, and Julia Kristeva. See *New French Feminisms*. Also see Judith Butler, *Bodies That Matter: On the Discursive Limits of "Sex"* (New York: Routledge, 1993); Elizabeth Grosz and Elspeth Probyn, eds., *Sexy Bodies: The Strange Carnalities of Feminism* (New York: Routledge, 1995); and my *HATREDS: Racialized and Sexualized Conflicts in the Twenty-first Century* (New York: Routledge, 1996) for a fuller set of citations about the female body.

174    4. Zillah Eisenstein, ed., *Capitalist Patriarchy and the Case for Socialist Feminism* (New York: Monthly Review Press, 1979). The actual date of publication was 1978, although the copyright mistakenly was dated 1979. I of course was working on this edited volume for several years before publication.

5. Zillah Eisenstein, *The Radical Future of Liberal Feminism* (Boston: Northeastern University Press, 1981).

6. Zillah Eisenstein, *The Female Body and the Law* (Berkeley: University of California Press, 1988).

7. Zillah Eisenstein, *The Color of Gender: Reimaging Democracy* (Berkeley: University of California Press, 1994).

8. Zillah Eisenstein, *Global Obscenities: Patriarchy, Capitalism, and the Lure of Cyberfantasy* (New York: New York University Press, 1998).

### Three. Theorizing a Breast Cancer Gene

1. Natalie Angier, *Woman: An Intimate Geography* (New York: Houghton Mifflin, 1999), 129.

2. Denise Grady, "Study Says Few Women Rue Preventive Breast Operation," *New York Times*, May 17, 1999, A14.

3. Margaret Lock and Deborah Gordon, eds., "Introduction," in *Biomedicine Examined* (Boston: Kluwer Academic Publisher, 1988), 4.

4. Nancy Krieger and Elizabeth Fee, "Man-Made Medicine and Women's Health: The Biopolitics of Sex/Gender and Race/Ethnicity," *International Journal of Health Services* 24, no. 2 (1994): 272.

5. Nikki vader Gaag, "Of Woman Born," *New Internationalist*, no. 303 (July 1998): 8.

6. I. Craig Henderson, "What Can a Woman Do about the Risk of Dying of Breast Cancer?" *Current Problems in Cancer* 14, no. 4 (July/August 1990): 166.

7. Liane Clorfene-Casten, *Breast Cancer: Poisons, Profits and Prevention* (Monroe, Maine: Common Courage Press, 1996), 13, 11.

8. Krieger and Fee, "Man-Made Medicine and Women's Health," 271.

9. Robert Proctor, *Cancer Wars: How Politics Shapes What We Do Know and Don't Know about Cancer* (New York: Basic Books, 1995), 255. Also see Jim Hightower, *There's Nothing in the Middle of the Road but Yellow Stripes and Dead Armadillos* (New York: HarperCollins, 1997).

10. Clorfene-Casten, *Breast Cancer*, 14.

11. For similar viewings of nature in science, see Ruth Bleier, *Science and Gender: A Critique of Biology and Its Theories about Women* (New York: Pergamon, 1984); Stephen Jay Gould, *The Flamingo's Smile: Reflections in Natural History* (New York: W. W. Norton, 1985); Marion Lowe and Ruth Hubbard, eds., *Woman's Nature: Rationalizations of Inequality* (New York: Pergamon Press, 1983); Carolyn Merchant, *The Death of Nature: Women, Ecology, and the Scientific Revolution*

(San Francisco: Harper and Row, 1980); and Janet Sayers, *Biological Politics: Feminist and Anti-feminist Perspectives* (New York: Tavistock, 1982). 175

12. Robert Arnot, *The Breast Cancer Prevention Diet: The Powerful Foods, Supplements, and Drugs That Can Save Your Life* (New York: Little, Brown, 1998), 19, 28; Susan Love with Karen Lindsey, *Dr. Susan Love's Breast Book* (Reading, Mass.: Addison-Wesley, 1990); Susan Love with Karen Lindsey, *Dr. Susan Love's Hormone Book: Making Informed Choices about Menopause* (New York: Random House, 1997); and Karen Stabiner, *To Dance with the Devil: The New War on Breast Cancer* (New York: Delacorte Press, 1997).

13. Jane Brody, "Round 3 in Cancer Battles: A 5 Year Drug Regimen," *New York Times*, May 11, 1999, F7.

14. Nancy Krieger, "Embodying Inequality: A Review of Concepts, Measures, and Methods for Studying Health Consequences of Discrimination," *International Journal of Health Services* 29, no. 2 (1999): 1295–1352.

15. Delease Wear and Lois LaCivita Nixon, *Literary Anatomies: Women's Bodies and Health in Literature* (Albany: State University of New York Press, 1994), 2.

16. Peter W. G. Wright, "Babyhood: The Social Construction of Infant Care as a Medical Problem in England in the Years around 1900," in *Biomedicine Examined*, ed. Margaret Lock and Deborah Gordon (Boston: Kluwer Academic Press, 1988), 301.

17. Nawal El Saadawi, *The Nawal El Saadawi Reader* (London: Zed, 1997), 54–58.

18. Sandra Steingraber, *Living Downstream: An Ecologist Looks at Cancer and the Environment* (New York: Addison-Wesley, 1997), 241, 251.

19. Proctor, *Cancer Wars*, 2.

20. Gilles Deleuze, *Foucault* (Minneapolis: University of Minnesota Press, 1988), 98, 123.

21. As quoted in Jennifer Myhre, "The Breast Cancer Movement: Seeing Beyond Consumer Activism," *Journal of the American Medical Women's Association* 54, no. 1 (winter 1999): 29–30. The full document is available from the Women's Community Cancer Project, c/o The Women's Center, 46 Pleasant St., Cambridge, MA 02139.

22. Quoting Donald Kennedy, then–Stanford University president, in Proctor, *Cancer Wars*, 4.

23. "The Truth about Breast Cancer—Final Part," *Rachel's Environment and Health Weekly*, no. 575 (December 4, 1997). Available from the Environmental Research Foundation, P.O. Box 5036, Annapolis, MD 21403; and on the internet at http://rachel.org/bulletin/bulletin.cfm?Issue_ID=545 or E-mail at erf@rachel.org or INFO@rachel.org. Also see Richard Doll and Richard Peto, "The Causes of Cancer: Quantitative Estimates of Avoidable Risks of Cancer in the U.S. Today," *Journal of the National Cancer Institute* 66, no. 6 (June 1981): 1191–1308.

176    24. Aldo Leopold, A Sand County Almanac, and Sketches Here and There (New York: Oxford University Press, 1949), 132.

### Four. Pluralized Environments in Black and White

1. This is stated in "A Ritual from the Clan of the Not-So-Many Breasted Women," which is a pamphlet of the Grail, an international women's organization committed to spiritual search, social action, and environmental sustainability. Information available from The Grail-Ancient Healing Project, 5401 Woodcrest Ave., Philadelphia, Pa. 19131; E-mail: upp.phila@juno.com.

2. World Cancer Research Fund in Association with American Institute for Cancer Research, Food, Nutrition, and the Prevention of Cancer: A Global Perspective (Washington, D.C.: American Institute for Cancer Research, 1997), 16, 55.

3. Peter Keating, "Protecting the Earth and the Poor," George 5, no. 5 (June 2000): 36. Also see Robert Bullard, ed., Confronting Environmental Racism: Voices from the Grassroots (Boston: South End Press, 1993).

4. Anna Volchkova, "Living with Chernobyl," Skipping Stones 11, no. 4 (November/December, 1998): 4.

5. Felicity Arbuthnot, "Poisoned Legacy," New Internationalist 316 (September 1999): 12, 13.

6. "No Spray Newz," no. 12, March 5, 2000. Available from the No Spray Coalition, New York, N.Y., at mitchelcohen@mindspring.com.

7. As discussed in Theo Colborn, Dianne Dumanoski, and John Peterson Myers, Our Stolen Future (New York: Dutton, 1996), 135–38.

8. Dan Fagin, Marianne Lavelle, and the Center for Public Integrity, Toxic Deception (New Jersey: Birch Lane Press, 1996), 138.

9. Ibid., xvii.

10. Colburn, Dumanoski, and Myers, Our Stolen Future, 138.

11. Marc Lappe, The Tao of Immunology (New York: Plenum Trade, 1997), 140, 162.

12. Andrea Martin, "Breast Cancer: Is It the Environment?" Ms. Magazine 10, no. 3 (April/May 2000): 48–52.

13. Rachel Carson, Silent Spring (New York: Houghton Mifflin, 1962), 15–17.

14. Ibid., 8.

15. "The Pops Treaty," Rachel's Environment and Health Weekly, no. 601 (June 4, 1998). Available from the Environmental Research Foundation, P.O. Box 5036, Annapolis, Md. 21403; and on the internet at erf@rachel.org; or E-mail at INFO@rachel.org.

16. Sandra Steingraber, Living Downstream: An Ecologist Looks at Cancer and the Environment (New York: Addison-Wesley, 1997), xv, 66.

17. World Cancer Research Fund, Food, Nutrition, and the Prevention of Cancer, 474.

18. Anne Underwood, Karen Springen, and Alisha Davis, "Cancer and Diet," 177
*Newsweek* 132, no. 22 (November 30, 1998): 60–66.

19. Jane Brody, "Diet Is Not a Panacea, but It Cuts Risk of Cancer," *New York Times*, December 1, 1998, F6.

20. Banoo Parpia, as quoted in *Choices: Newsletter of the Ithaca Breast Cancer Alliance*, no. 16 (Fall 1998): 5. I am indebted to several conversations with Banoo Parpia, Chief Coordinator of the Cornell-China Oxford Project.

21. Robert Arnot, *The Breast Cancer Prevention Diet* (New York: Little, Brown, 1998).

22. Robert Proctor, *Cancer Wars* (New York: Basic Books, 1995), 16.

23. "Toxic Turnaround," *Rachel's Environment and Health Weekly*, no. 602 (June 11, 1998).

24. Frederick Noronha, "Warning: Time Is Running Out for Asia's Forests," *New Internationalist*, no. 303 (July 1998): 5.

25. Fred Magdoff, John Bellamy Foster, and Frederick H. Buttel, *Monthly Review*, "Introduction," Special Issue: "Hungry Profit," 50, no. 3 (July/August 1998): 5.

26. John Bellamy Foster and Fred Magdoff, "Liebig, Marx, and the Depletion of Soil Fertility: Relevance for Today's Agriculture," *Monthly Review* 50, no. 3 (July/August 1998): 32.

27. John Bellamy Foster, "The Scale of Our Ecological Crisis", *Monthly Review Press* 49, no. 11 (April 1998): 5–15.

28. "Environmental Justice in Louisiana," *Rachel's Environment and Health Weekly* no. 615 (September 10, 1998). Available at listserv@rachel.org or from the Environmental Research Foundation at P.O. Box 5036, Annapolis, Md. 21403.

29. Jean Hardisty and Ellen Leopold, "Cancer and Poverty: Double Jeopardy for Women," in *Myths about the Powerless: Contesting Social Inequalities*, ed. M. B. Wykes et al. (Philadelphia: Temple University Press, 1996): 220.

30. Mary Anglin, "Working from the Inside Out: Implications of Breast Cancer Activism for Biomedical Policies and Practices," *Social Science Medicine* 44, no. 9 (1997): 1407, 1411–12.

31. See Nancy Krieger's statement "Racial Discrimination and Health: An Epidemiologist's Perspective" for the *President's Cancer Panel Meeting: The Meaning of Race in Science*, April 9, 1997.

32. Nancy Krieger et al., "Race/Ethnicity, Social Class, and Prevalence of Breast Cancer Prognostic BioMarkers: A Study of White, Black, and Asian Women in the San Francisco Bay Area," *Ethnicity and Disease* 7 (Spring/Summer 1997): 137, 138.

33. Nancy Krieger, "Social Class and the Black/White Crossover in the Age-Specific Incidence of Breast Cancer: A Study Linking Census-Derived Data to Population-Based Registry Records", *American Journal of Epidemiology* 131, no. 5 (1990): 804, 805, 810, 812.

34. As quoted in Alexis Jetter, "Breast Cancer in Blacks Spurs Hunt for Answers," *New York Times*, February 22, 2000, F7.

178     35. From my interview and meeting with Ngina Lythcott, Mailman School of Public Health, Columbia University, May 25, 2000.

36. "The Long Island Solid Waste Crisis and Toxic Chemical Exposure-Induced Breast Cancer Report," delivered before the Subcommittee on Environment of the Committee on Science, Space and Technology, U.S. House of Representatives, 102 Congress, May 8, 1992. Report no. 138. Available from the U.S. Government Printing Office, Washington, D.C. 20402.

37. Marc Lappe, *Chemical Deception* (San Francisco: Sierra Club Books, 1991).

38. Samuel Epstein, *The Politics of Cancer* (San Francisco: Sierra Club Books, 1978).

39. Ralph Moss, *The Cancer Industry* (New York: Paragon House, 1989): 417.

40. Liane Clorfene-Casten, *Breast Cancer: Poisons, Profits and Prevention* (Monroe, Maine: Common Courage Press, 1996).

41. Moss, *Cancer Industry*, 389, 394.

42. Judy Brady, "Follow the Money," paper delivered at the Second World Conference on Breast Cancer, Ottawa, Canada, July 26-31, 1999.

43. Jim Hightower, *There's Nothing in the Middle of the Road but Yellow Stripes and Dead Armadillos* (New York: HarperCollins, 1997); and "The Truth about Breast Cancer," *Rachel's Environment and Health Weekly*, Part 2, no. 572, November 13, 1997.

44. James Bennett and Thomas DiLorenzo, *CancerScam* (New Brunswick, N.J.: Transaction, 1998), 2, 3.

45. Clorfene-Casten, *Breast Cancer*, 262.

46. Proctor, *Cancer Wars*, 36, 45.

47. Ibid., 8.

48. Edith Efron, *The Apocalyptics: Cancer and the Big Lie* (New York: Simon & Schuster, 1984), 428.

49. John W. Gofman, *Preventing Breast Cancer: The Story of a Major, Proven, Preventable Cause of This Disease* (San Francisco: Committee for Nuclear Responsibility, 1996), 5.

50. Steingraber, *Living Downstream*, 11.

51. Epstein, *The Politics of Cancer*, 2.

52. Ibid., 40, 63, 65.

53. For information related to the BRCA1 and 2 gene, contact "Genetic Testing for Risk of Breast and Ovarian Cancer," Myriad Genetic Laboratories, 320 Wakara Way, Salt Lake City, Utah 84108, E-mail: BRACA@myriad.com; or Hadassah, Domestic Agenda, 50 West 58 St., New York, N.Y. 10019. Also see Jane Brody, "Disclosure of How a Gene Causes Breast Cancer," *New York Times*, August 14, 1998, A14.

54. Epstein, *Politics of Cancer*, 59, 61-63, 259, 260,

55. Ibid., 112.

## Five. Radicalizing the Pink-Ribboned Breast for Us All 179

1. Zillah Eisenstein, *The Female Body and the Law* (Berkeley: University of California Press, 1988).

2. Carolyn Latteier, *Breasts: The Women's Perspective on an American Obsession* (New York: Haworth Press, 1998).

3. I use the terms masculinist and patriarchal interchangeably in my text. Both focus attention on the sex/gender system of male privilege as both an ideational and a structural system.

4. "Tumor Suppressor Genes—Guardians of Our Cells," Fact Sheet no. 6, from the *Program on Breast Cancer and Environmental Risk Factors in New York State*, December, 1997, 2–3. Available at 110 Rice Hall, Cornell University, Ithaca, N.Y. 14853. Also see http://www.cfe.cornell.edu/bcerf/

5. Susan Love, *Dr. Susan Love's Breast Book*, 2d ed. (New York: Addison-Wesley, 1995), 165–187.

6. Barbara Katz Rothman, *Genetic Maps and Human Imagination* (New York: Norton, 1998), 151.

7. Love, *Dr. Susan Love's Breast Book*, 186.

8. Sandra Steingraber, "Lifestyles Don't Kill. Carcinogens in Air, Food and Water Do: Imagining Political Responses to Cancer," in *Cancer as a Woman's Issue*, ed. Midge Stocker, (Chicago: Third Side Press, 1991), 91–102.

9. Nancy Krieger and Elizabeth Fee, "Man-Made Medicine and Women's Health: The Biopolitics of Sex/Gender and Race/Ethnicity," *International Journal of Health Services* 24, no. 2 (1994): 265–283.

10. Robert Bazell, *Her-2: The Making of Hercepton, A Revolutionary Treatment for Breast Cancer* (New York: Random House, 1998), 51.

11. See: Love, *Dr. Susan Love's Breast Book*; and Karen Stabiner, *To Dance with the Devil: The New War on Breast Cancer* (New York: Delacorte Press, 1997).

12. Margaret Lock and Patricia Kaufert, eds., *Pragmatic Women and Body Politics* (Cambridge: Cambridge University Press, 1998). Also see Susan Sherwin, coordinator of the Feminist Health Care Ethics Research Network, et al., *The Politics of Women's Health* (Philadelphia: Temple University Press, 1998).

13. Michelle Saint Germain and Aluce Longman, "Resignation and Resourcefulness: Older Hispanic Women's Responses to Breast Cancer," in *Wings of Gauze: Women of Color and the Experience of Health and Illness*, eds. Barbara Bair and Susan Cayleff, (Detroit: Wayne State University Press, 1993), 269.

14. Teresa Jacok, Leslie Spieth, and Nolan Penn, "Breast Cancer, Breast Self Examination, and African-American Women," in Bair and Cayleff, *Wings of Gauze*, 244.

15. "Childhood Life Events and the Risk of Breast Cancer," in *Breast Cancer and Environmental Risk Factors*, Fact Sheet no. 8, March 1998, p. 1. Available from BCERF.

180      16. "Do We Need to be Concerned About Environmental Chemicals and Breast Cancer?" *The Ribbon*, 2, no. 3 (fall, 1997): 1, 3. Available from BCERF.

17. I. Craig Henderson, "What Can a Woman Do about the Risk of Dying of Breast Cancer?" *Current Problems in Cancer* 14, no 4 (July/August 1990): 168.

18. "Reducing the Risk for Breast Cancer," *The Ribbon*, 1, no. 2 (fall, 1996): 1, 3.

19. I. Craig Henderson, "Risk Factors for Breast Cancer Development," *Cancer* 71, no. 6, supplement (March 15, 1993): 2127.

20. Bazell, *Her-2*, 7.

21. Love, *Dr. Susan Love's Breast Book*, 183.

22. I. Craig Henderson, "What Can a Woman Do about the Risk of Dying of Breast Cancer?" *Current Problems in Cancer* 14, no. 4 (July/August 1990): 165.

23. John Gofman, *Preventing Breast Cancer: The Story of a Major, Proven, Preventable Cause of This Disease* (San Francisco: Committee for Nuclear Responsibility, 1996), 2. Also see Richard Doll and Richard Peto, "The Causes of Cancer: Quantitative Estimates of Avoidable Risks of Cancer in the U.S. Today," *Journal of the National Cancer Institute* 66, no. 6 (June 1981): 1191–1309.

24. Statistics from the National Cancer Institute, and quoted in "Breast Cancer and Environmental Risk Factors—Questions, Answers, and Information," *The Ribbon* 1, no. 1 (spring 1996): 1.

25. "Understanding Breast Cancer Rates," Fact Sheet no. 3, BCERF, August 1997, p. 2. Available from BCERF, Cornell University.

26. "Intergenerational Education: Starting Early to Reduce Breast Cancer Risk," *The Ribbon* 2, no. 2 (spring 1997): 1.

27. "The Truth about Breast Cancer," *Rachel's Environment and Health Weekly*, no. 571, (November 6, 1997). Available from the Environmental Research Foundation, P.O. Box 5036, Annapolis, Md. 21403; and on the internet at erf@rachel.org; or E-mail at INFO@rachel.org

28. Liane Clorfene-Casten, *Breast Cancer: Poisons, Profits and Prevention* (Monroe, Maine: Common Courage Press, 1996), 113.

29. Robert Proctor, *Cancer Wars* (New York: Basic Books, 1995), 255.

30. "The Truth about Breast Cancer."

31. Nancy Krieger, Mary S. Wolff, Robert A. Hiatt, Marilyn Rivera, Joseph Vogelman, and Norman Orentreich, "Breast Cancer and Serum Organochlorines: A Prospective Study among White, Black, and Asian Women," *Journal of the National Cancer Institute* 86, no. 8 (April 20, 1994): 592.

32. J. W. Berg, "Clinical Implications of Risk Factors for Breast Cancer," *Cancer* 53 (1984): 589.

33. Nancy Krieger, "Exposure, Susceptibility, and Breast Cancer Risk," *Breast Cancer Research and Treatment* 205 (1989): 208. Also see Nancy Krieger, Stephen Van Den Eeden, David Zava, and Akiko Okamoto, "Race/Ethnicity, Social Class, and Prevalence of Breast Cancer Prognostic Biomarkers: A Study of White, Black, and Asian Women in the San Francisco Bay Area," *Ethnicity and Disease* 7

(spring/summer 1997): 137–49.

34. Krieger, "Exposure, Susceptibility, and Breast Cancer Risk," 208–10, 211, 212–14.

35. Ibid.: also see her "Epidemiology and the Web of Causation: Has Anyone Seen the Spider?" *Social Science Medicine* 39, no. 7 (1994): 887–903; and "Inequality, Diversity, and Health: Thoughts on 'Race/Ethnicity' and 'Gender,'" *Journal of American Medical Women's Association* 51, no. 4 (August/October 1996): 133–36.

36. Proctor, *Cancer Wars*, 240.

37. Ibid., 223.

38. Clorfene-Casten, *Breast Cancer*, 15, 16.

39. George Crile, *The Breast Cancer Controversy: What Women Should Know About* (New York: Macmillan, 1973), 122.

40. Henderson, "What Can a Woman Do?" 172.

41. I am indebted to discussions with Banoo Parpia, researcher on "The China Project," Cornell University. Also see T. J. A. Key et al., "Sex Hormones in Women in Rural China and in Britain," *British Journal of Cancer* 62 (1990): 631–36.

42. Thanks to Anna Marie Smith for discussion of this point.

43. Patricia Kaufert, "Menopause as Process or Event: The Creation of Definitions in Biomedicine," in *Biomedicine Examined*, eds. Margaret Lock and Deborah Gordon (Boston: Kluwer Academic Pub., 1988), 340.

44. Margaret Lock, "The Politics of Mid-Life and Menopause", in *Knowledge, Power, and Practice*, eds. Shirley Lindenbaum and Margaret Lock (Berkeley: University of California Press, 1993) 332.

45. Ibid., 350–52.

46. Richard Stevens, Bary Wilson, and Larry Anderson, *The Metatonin Hypothesis* (Columbus, Ohio: Battelle Press, 1997), 9.

47. Data are available from Hadassah, The Women's Zionist Organization of America, The Women's Breast Cancer Education Program, 50 West 58th Street, New York, N.Y. 10019. http://www.hadassah.org

48. "Estrogen and Breast Cancer Risk: What Is the Relationship?" Fact Sheet no. 9, March 1998, BCERF, p. 3.

49. Clorfene-Casten, *Breast Cancer*, 101.

50. Janette Sherman, "Tamoxifen and Prevention of Breast Cancer," *Toxicology and Industrial Health* 14, no. 4 (1998): 485, 495. Also see her *Life's Delicate Balance* (New York: Taylor and Francis, 2000).

51. Gina Kolata and Lawrence Fisher, "Drugs to Fight Breast Cancer Near Approval," *New York Times*, September 3, 1998, A1.

52. Robert Pear, "Preventive Use of Tamoxifen Is Allowed", *New York Times*, October 30, 1998, A27.

53. Robert Arnot, *The Breast Cancer Prevention Diet* (New York: Little Brown, 1998), 10; and Bazell, *Her-2*, 26.

54. The study, known as the Hormone Replacement Therapy trial of the

182  Women's Health Initiative, is the first large-scale clinical trial to test the efficacy of ERT for the heart in postmenopausal women. Gina Kolata, "Estrogen Tied to Slight Increase in Risk to Heart, a Study Hints," *New York Times*, April 4, 2000, A1.

55. Kolata and Fisher, "Drugs to Fight Breast Cancer Near Approval," A1.

56. Frances Visco's NBCC statement for immediate release, April 7, 1998.

57. "Tamoxifen for Prevention," report issued by the National Women's Health Network, April 1998, p. 75. Available from 514 Tenth St. N.W., Suite 400, Washington, D.C. 20004.

58. Ibid., 15.

59. M. H. Gail et al., "Weighing the Risks and Benefits of Tamoxifen Treatment for Preventing Breast Cancer," *Journal of the National Cancer Institute*, November 3, 1999, 1829–46. Also see http://www.FDA.gov; and www.nsabp.pitt.edu.

60. Cindy Pearson, "Tamoxifen for Healthy Women: Risk Reduction for Whom?" *Network News*, January/February 2000, 5.

61. Pear, "Preventive Use of Tamoxifen," A27.

62. Esther Dreifuss-Kattan, *Cancer Stories: Creativity and Repair* (Hillsdale, N.J.: Analytic Press, 1990); Deborah Hobler Kahane, *No Less a Woman* (Almeda, Calif.: Hunter House, 1990); Joan Nestle, *A Fragile Union* (San Francisco: Cleis Press, 1998); and Marianne Paget, *A Complex Sorrow* (Philadelphia: Temple University Press, 1993).

63. The Boston Women's Health Book Collective, *Our Bodies/Ourselves* (New York: Simon & Schuster, 1976).

64. See the recent breast cancer literature for a fuller discussion of many of these issues. Lois Tschetter Hjelmstad, *Fine Black Lines* (Denver: Mulberry Hill Press, 1993, 1998); Ellen Leopold, *A Darker Ribbon* (Boston: Beacon Press, 1999); Susan Moss, *Keep Your Breasts* (Los Angeles: Source Publications, 1994, 1998); Laura Potts, ed., *Ideologies of Breast Cancer* (New York: St. Martins Press, 2000); and Hilda Raz, ed., *Living on the Margins* (New York: Persea Books, 1999).

65. Patricia Kaufert, "Women, Resistance and the Breast Cancer Movement", in Lock and Kaufert, *Pragmatic Women and Body Politics*, 287–310.

66. Mary Anglin, "Working from the Inside Out: Implications of Breast Cancer Activism for Biomedical Policies and Practices," *Social Science Medicine* 44, no. 9, (1997): 1403–15.

67. Rose Kushner, *Why Me?* (Philadelphia: Saunders Press, 1982), republished as *Alternatives: New Developments in the War on Breast Cancer* (New York: Warner Books, 1984).

68. National Breast Cancer Coalition: www.natlbcc.org

69. Materials are available from WCCP, c/o Women's Center, 46 Pleasant St., Cambridge, Mass. 02139

70. I wish to thank Andrea Martin for her telephone conversations with me, in May 2000, and for the materials she made so readily available.

71. Maren Klawiter, "Racing for the Cure: Walking Women and Toxic Touring:   183
Mapping Cultures of Action with the Bay Area Terrain of Breast Cancer," *Social
Problems* 46, no. 1 (1999): 104–26.

## Six. Returning to Feminism through the Locale of the Breast

1. Michel Foucault, *The History of Sexuality*, vol. 1 (New York: Pantheon Books,
1978).

2. There is a huge feminist literature discussing these issues. For particularly
provocative discussions, see Judith Butler, *Bodies That Matter* (New York: Routledge, 1993); Elisabeth Grosz and Elspeth Probyn, *Sexy Bodies* (New York: Routledge, 1995); and Eve Kosofsky Sedgwick, *Tendencies* (Durham: Duke University
Press, 1993).

3. As quoted in Andrew Morton, *Monica's Story* (New York: St. Martin's Press,
1999), 252, 263, 279.

4. Gwendolyn Mink, *Hostile Environment* (Ithaca: Cornell University Press,
2000).

5. Kathie Sarachild, ed., *Feminist Revolution* (New Paltz, N.Y.: Redstockings,
1975).

6. For a sampling of this huge literature, see bell hooks, *Talking Back* (Boston:
South End Press, 1989); Barbara Smith, ed., *Home Girls: A Black Feminist Anthol-
ogy* (New York: Kitchen Table Women of Color Press, 1983); Patricia Williams, *The
Alchemy of Race and Rights* (Cambridge: Harvard University Press, 1991).

7. Richard Dyer, *WHITE* (New York: Routledge, 1997); and David Roediger,
*Black on White* (New York: Schocken, 1998).

8. Joel Williamson, *New People, Miscegenation and Mulattoes in the U.S.*
(Baton Rouge: Louisiana State University Press, 1995), 57, 63, 95. Also see Angela
Davis, "Reflections on the Black Woman's Role in the Community of Slaves," *Black
Scholar* 3, no. 4 (December 1971): 3-15, and her *Women, Race, and Class* (New York:
Random House, 1981); Edward Ball, *Slaves in the Family* (New York: Ballantine,
1998); and John Hope Franklin and Loren Schweninger, *Runaway Slaves* (New
York: Oxford University Press, 1991).

9. Shirlee Taylor Haizlip, *The Sweeter the Juice* (New York: Simon & Schuster,
1994), 30, 15.

10. Ibid., 138, 139.

11. As stated in James Bennet, "Clinton Admits Lewinsky Liaison to Jury; Tells
Nation 'It was Wrong,' But Private," *New York Times*, August 16, 1998, A1.

12. Orlando Patterson, "What Is Freedom without Privacy?" *New York Times*,
September 15, 1998, p. A27.

13. Wendy Wasserstein, "Hillary Clinton's Muddled Legacy," *New York Times*,
August 25, 1998, p. A17.

184     14. John Broder, "On an Island Retreat, a Time for Healing," *New York Times*, August 19, 1998, A23.

15. Gwendolyn Mink, "Should the Truth Faze Feminists?" *New York Times*, August 18, 1998, A25.

16. Maureen Dowd, "Saturday Night Bill," *New York Times*, August 19, 1998, A31.

17. See my *HATREDS* (New York: Routledge, 1996) for a full accounting of this argument.

18. Sandra Steingraber, "Why the Precautionary Principle? A Meditation on Polyvinyl Chloride (PVC) and the Breasts of Mothers," in *Rachel's Environment and Health Weekly*, no. 658 (July 8, 1999). Available from the Environmental Research Foundation, P.O. Box 5036, Annapolis, Md. 21403; and on the internet at *erf@rachel.org*; or E-mail at *INFO@rachel.org*.

19. Sandra Steingraber, "Protecting the First Environment: Thoughts on Toxic Chemicals and Pregnancy," paper, January 2000.

**Seven. Taking the Breast to the Globe**

1. I have been involved in this dialogue for a quarter-century now. This discussion starts from the many places it has been located over these years and cannot be fully understood in the here and now. Please see my *The Color of Gender: Reimaging Democracy* (Berkeley: University of California Press, 1994); *HATREDS: Racialized and Sexualized Conflicts in the Twenty-first Century* (New York: Routledge, 1996); and *Global Obscenities: Patriarchy, Capitalism, and the Lure of Cyberfantasy* (New York: New York University Press, 1998) for tracing these issues within the historical contexts defining them. One will find appropriate bibliographical citation in order to more completely study the issues and authors involved.

2. Nawal El Saadawi, *The Nawal El Saadawi Reader* (London: Zed Press, 1977), 18.

3. Much of my thinking here is indebted to conversations with Rosalind Petchesky as we have explored the necessity for feminists of dealing with issues of global capital *and* governance. We continue to explore the limits and the necessity of local politics.

4. Rosalind Petchesky, "Reproductive and Sexual Rights, Social Development and Globalization: Charting the Course of Transnational Women's NGO's," *United Nations Research Institute for Social Development*, 2000; her unpublished "Global Citizenship and Women's Power: A Critical Reassessment," Stites Lecture in Social Science, delivered at the University of Washington, Seattle, February 2000; and Petchesky and Karen Judd, eds., *Negotiating Reproductive Rights: Women's Perspectives across Countries and Cultures* (New York: St. Martin's Press, 1998). Also see Kalpana Ram, "Na Shariram Nadhi, My Body Is Mine: The Urban Women's Health

Movement in India and Its Negotiation of Modernity," *Women's Studies Interna-* 185
*tional Forum* 21, no. 6 (1998): 86–112.

5. David Rieff, *Los Angeles: Capital of the Third World* (New York: Simon &
Schuster, 1991).

6. The term *glocal* is also used by Paul Virilio in his *Open Sky* (London: Verso
Press, 1997), 135.

7. Women's Environment and Development Organization (WEDO), "A Gender Approach for the WTO," available at http://www.wedo.org.

8. Robert Edgar, "Jubilee 2000; Paying Our Debts," *Nation* 270, no. 16 (April 24,
2000): 20.

9. Sheryl Gay Stolberg, "'Epidemic of Oral Disease' Is Found in Poor," *New
York Times*, May 26, 2000, A15.

10. U.N. Report of the Commission on Human Rights, "Human Rights of
Women and Violence against Them," April 12, 2000, press release. Available at
http://www.unog.ch/news2/documents/newsen/cn0036e.html; and Donald G. Mc-
Neil Jr., "Drug Companies and Third World: A Case Study in Neglect," *New York
Times*, May 21, 2000, A1. Also see Hans d'Orville, *United Nations Development Program (UNDP) and the Communication Revolution: Communications and Knowl-
edge-Based Technologies for Sustainable Human Development*, at http://www.undp
.org/comm/techn.htm, especially chapters 2 and 4.

11. Quoted from the report "Vital Signs 1998," conducted by World Watch Institute, a Washington-based environmental group, in Barbara Crossette, "A New Measure of Disparities: Poor Sanitation in Internet Era," *New York Times*, May 12, 1998,
A11; and United Nations Development Programme information, at http://www.undp
.org.

12. See the MADRE literature on cuba, especially the Share Hope Campaign,
at http://www.MADRE.org.

13. Ibid.

14. Denise Grady, "Trapped at the South Pole, Doctor Becomes a Patient," *New
York Times*, July 13, 1999, A1.

15. World Conference on Breast Cancer, Ottawa, Canada, July 26–31, 1999.
Corporate sponsors were Kodak, Scotiabank, Canadian Dairy Products, Biomira,
Canadian Airlines, and Corel.

16. Andaiye, "Cancer and Power," paper delivered at the World Conference on
Breast Cancer, Ottawa, Canada, July 26–31, 1999.

17. See my chapter "Feminism of the North and West for Export," in *HA-
TREDS*.

18. Jeffrey Bartholet, "The Plague Years," *Newsweek* 135, no. 3 (January 17, 2000):
32.

19. Sandra Steingraber, "Why the Precautionary Principle? A Meditation on

186 Polyvinyl Chloride (PVC) and the Breasts of Mothers," *Rachel's Environment and Health Weekly*, no. 658 (July 8, 1999). Available from the Environmental Research Foundation, P.O. Box 5036, Annapolis, MD 21403; and on the internet at http://rachel.org/bulletin/bulletin.cfm?Issue_ID=1515 or E-mail at erf@rachel.org or INFO@rachel.org.

20. Carlos Fuentes, "Introduction," in Frida Kahlo, *The Diary of Frida Kahlo: An Intimate Self-Portrait* (New York: H. N. Abrams, 1995), 16.

# INDEX

# Index